Advance Praise for *In Our Words*

"Psychogenic non-epileptic seizures (PNES) are a common malady that is frequently misunderstood. Those with this disorder are often belittled by both health care practitioners and the general public. This collection of self-descriptions from people with PNES are eye awakening and help significantly to dispel many inaccurate myths. They provide a window into the many facets and presentations of this disorder and how it can be incapacitating. Testimonies to therapeutic success are encouraging and instructive. My congratulations to the authors for collecting these personal recounts and to the participants for their honesty and integrity."

—John J. Barry, MD
Professor of Neuropsychiatry
Stanford University Medical Center
Stanford, CA

"This collection of testimonies by people with Psychogenic Non-epileptic Seizures (PNES) (and their family members) from around the world is an immensely valuable addition to the Brainstorms series. The international nature of the experiences and the common themes expressed so honestly by the writers should reassure others with PNES that they are not alone in their attempts to understand their experiences and deal with the many challenges to which having PNES gives rise. The experiences described make this book a crucial aid in communicating to family and friends what the person with PNES is going through. For healthcare professionals this book is a "must read"-understanding the breadth of people's difficult experiences is essential to the provision of good patient-centred care. If only this book had been available sooner!"

—Laura H. Goldstein, PhD, MPhil
Professor of Clinical Neuropsychology
Institute of Psychiatry Psychology and Neuroscience
King's College
London, UK

"Bravo to all the people who have courageously shared their individual experiences of dissociative (non-epileptic) seizures in this unique book. From bewilderment, shame and humiliation to understanding, treatment and hope—it is essential reading for patients and health professionals."

—Dr. Jon Stone
Consultant Neurologist and Honorary Reader in Neurology
University of Edinburgh
Edinburgh, UK

In Our Words

In Our Words

Personal Accounts of Living with Non-Epileptic Seizures

Markus Reuber, MD

Academic Neurology Unit
University of Sheffield and Department of Neurology
Sheffield Teaching Hospitals NHS Foundation Trust
Sheffield, United Kingdom

Gregg Rawlings, PhD

Academic Unit of Elderly Care and Rehabilitation
Bradford Teaching Hospitals NHS Foundation Trust
Bradford, United Kingdom

Steven C. Schachter, MD

Departments of Neurology,
Beth Israel Deaconess Medical Center,
Massachusetts General Hospital, and
Harvard Medical School
Boston, USA

OXFORD
UNIVERSITY PRESS

OXFORD
UNIVERSITY PRESS

Oxford University Press is a department of the University of Oxford. It furthers
the University's objective of excellence in research, scholarship, and education
by publishing worldwide. Oxford is a registered trade mark of Oxford University
Press in the UK and certain other countries.

Published in the United States of America by Oxford University Press
198 Madison Avenue, New York, NY 10016, United States of America.

© Oxford University Press 2018

CIP data is on file at the Library of Congress
ISBN 978–0–19–062277–0

1 3 5 7 9 8 6 4 2
Printed by Webcom Inc., Canada

CONTENTS

FOREWORD

Siri Hustvedt

Taken as a whole, the testimonies in this book, written by people who suffer or have suffered from psychogenic non-epileptic seizures (PNES), sound a call to action. PNES is neither a rare disorder nor a new one. The medical literature on the illness is many centuries old. In 1682, the renowned English doctor Thomas Sydenham described what was then called "hysteria" as a "chameleon-like" disease and linked it to the patient's "antecedent sorrows." In the late nineteenth century, the French neurologist Jean-Martin Charcot proposed that, unlike epilepsy, "hysterical seizures" are caused by a "dynamic or functional lesion" in the brain that leaves no trace during autopsy. Charcot classified the illness as neurological, not psychiatric, and he further argued that it could be initiated by a shock or trauma in the patient's life. Although the name has changed over time and diagnostic categories have shifted, PNES, along with other functional neurological disorders, has long hovered in the bewildering and discomfiting borderland between physiological and psychological, between neurology and psychiatry, between body and mind.

Although many physicians pay lip service to the idea that psyche and soma cannot be viewed as separate entities, that the mind does not float over the body as a cloud drifts above the earth, that the brain is crucial to generating what we think of as mental states, many continue to regard patients who have been given a diagnosis of PNES with suspicion. Patients in this volume report being told by doctors that their condition isn't "real," or that "it's all in your head." One patient writes, "I was diagnosed by a neurologist with a purely 'psychological' disorder, nothing to do with the brain, and given a pamphlet. I cried in the toilet of the hospital for an hour at my unexpected diagnosis of madness" (see Chapter 2). Another patient tells us, "I am a nurse, and I have worked on a neuroscience ward. We have a patient whose mum has pseudoseizures, and the nurses always mock her or say she is weird and fakes seizures—these are professionals and even they don't understand it" (see Chapter 15).

Sadly, the behavior of the neurologist and the nursing staff in these accounts is not atypical. Although the professionals involved are not necessarily driven by cruelty, their callous behavior is born of a mixture of prejudice, misunderstanding, ignorance, and embarrassment. Non-epileptic seizures have puzzled physicians since the Greeks, and despite important research uncovering the brain regions and processes involved in PNES, no one truly understands how they occur. Although it is difficult for many doctors to admit ignorance, I think they should be honest with patients that much remains to be discovered about the nature of these seizures. Scientific humility is crucial. But it is also vital for doctors to tell their patients that these gaps in knowledge do not mean PNES are immune to therapy.

As a person who had four dramatic, non-epileptic shaking episodes between 2006 and 2007—three while speaking in public and one in private while climbing a mountain far ahead of my husband and a friend—I am well acquainted with the startling sensation of losing control of one's own body. It's shocking. The first time I went into spasms, I was speaking at a memorial event for my father, a fact that seemed highly significant at the time and still does. I wrote a book about my symptom called *The Shaking Woman or A History of My Nerves,* a wide-ranging investigation of my attacks from multiple disciplinary points of view, including medical history, philosophy, psychiatry, neurology, and neuroscience. I consider myself lucky, not only because I can count my shaking events on one hand and I have not suffered from seizures since, but also because for years before I had my first attack, I had been immersed in the mind-body problem. My symptom presented itself as an interesting "object" for me to explore as a writer and thinker. I am excruciatingly conscious of the fact that this makes my story different from those of most people in this book.

PNES are not caused by the type of abnormal electrical activity seen with epileptic seizures or a visible lesion in the brain, and it is essential for doctors to distinguish them from other possible diagnoses to avoid unnecessary and dangerous treatments or interventions that will make the patient's condition even worse. Further, there are those who have both epileptic and non-epileptic seizures. This surely complicates the task of diagnosis, and yet, as is obvious from some of the narratives compiled in this book, suffering from epilepsy is not "more real" than suffering from PNES. Human beings may be incapacitated by both illnesses. *All suffering is real.* None of us dies from PNES, however. And people do die of intractable epileptic seizures and other wasting neurological diseases, so it is crucial that patients understand that receiving a diagnosis of PNES is in many ways a "good" diagnosis. Indeed, a number of people describe the immense relief they felt after finally having a name for what was wrong with them.

What every reader will discover in this book is how various the illness is, and how, despite certain commonalities, every person's experience is different from every other's. The eighteenth-century physician Thomas Sydenham was right— there is a chameleon-like quality to these disorders. The stigma attached to what is currently called PNES is greater now than it was when the man called the English Hippocrates was writing, however. Patients today must contend not only with the misery of their attacks but also with the incomprehension of professionals in the medical community and the wider public. When coupled with the illness itself, this brutal prejudice conspires to make patients feel even lonelier and more helpless.

Speaking out about one's experience with PNES is not a cure, but it may be the beginning of a person's path to gaining a greater sense of agency in his or her life, which I believe is also key to alleviating the symptoms. Some patients in this book acknowledge the benefits they have received from working with psychiatrists who are trained in the illness. My favorite summary of a cure is this one: "Through my treatment for neurological functional disorder with my fabulous psychiatrist, I am now seizure free" (see Chapter 11). This patient does not provide the details of that treatment, but it is safe to conclude the healing took place in an atmosphere of mutual respect and recognition rather than one of suspicion. People with PNES can get better. They can be helped, but only if they are accorded the dignity their many stories of suffering deserve.

Siri Hustvedt, PhD
Novelist, Essayist, and Lecturer in Psychiatry
at Weill Cornell Medical College of Cornell University, NY, USA

FOREWORD

Lorna Myers

Those who live with psychogenic non-epileptic seizures (PNES) bear a heavy load. For whatever reasons, they have developed episodes that look very much like epileptic seizures. These can range from extreme, whole-body paralysis to violent thrashing of some or all limbs, can last from seconds to hours, can cause injuries, and often result in the loss of basic privileges, such as driving, holding a job, or attending classes. Too often, precursors to the onset of seizures are traumatic in nature, with about eighty percent of those diagnosed with PNES reporting one or more severe psychological traumas in their lifetime, meaning that they have a much higher incidence of severe trauma than we see in the general population.

Sadly, the final blow is frequently dealt by those who are charged with caring for the patient: the health care professionals. PNES is still very much an orphan disorder in the field of health care, with medical doctors understanding PNES as a mental disorder (which is accurate) and, therefore, not their business (which is not accurate). On the other hand, mental health professionals tend to view PNES as something that resembles a medical disorder (which is true) and, therefore, not psychological nor amenable to psychotherapy (which is not true). PNES reflect a complex health condition that bridges both the physical and the psychological, and as such, it demands a multi-disciplinary approach. However, because of the misconceptions health professionals hold, patients can end up bouncing between medical (e.g., neurology and emergency medical departments) and mental health (e.g., psychiatry and psychology) agencies, all the while becoming more frustrated and hopeless, and worsening the chances of recovery. Health professionals also become frustrated, feel helpless, and may increasingly respond to the patient with dismissive or even hostile attitudes and behaviors. As could be expected, if the health professionals don't understand the severity and respect those with the condition, the general public cannot be expected to do any better. This pejorative attitude toward people with PNES is probably one of the most hurtful and distressing aspects of the condition—not only is the person seriously ill and suffering, but empathy and genuine efforts to help are mostly absent.

I have been evaluating and treating patients diagnosed with PNES for over fifteen years now. PNES intrigued me from day one, from the very first patient I met in the epilepsy unit so many years back. And I can say that the years spent working with PNES have only deepened my interest in this condition and made me eager to try to find ways to better understand and treat it.

I have been "speaking" to persons with PNES for many years in my therapy office. However, in the last few years, especially with the advent of social media, my ability to "speak" with those living with PNES has changed quite dramatically. If I trace how this happened, I think that the initial shift began after I published a book for patients, *Psychogenic Non-epileptic Seizures: A Guide*. My goal for that book was to speak to those living with PNES who were not making it to my office. At the end of the book, I included my email address so that I might have a conversation with some of the readers. I began to receive messages and requests from across the United States and abroad. Soon after, the next reasonable step was to host a website and a blog (both at http://blog.nonepilepticseizures.com/), as well as a PNES Facebook page called *Psychological Non-Epileptic Seizures*. These multiple means of communication created a most valuable portal that has allowed me to communicate extensively and regularly with those touched by PNES (patients, loved ones, professionals). Because I have spoken with so many in these ways over the last few years, I am especially thrilled to see this PNES Brainstorms book published. It compiles accurately and poignantly the experience of those living with PNES across the globe, exquisitely showing the uniqueness of PNES in each individual along with the universality of the disorder, regardless of the continent or the country in which the person diagnosed with PNES lives.

As I read one testimony after another in this PNES Brainstorms edition, I felt great satisfaction and excitement at how impeccably the accounts have captured the multilayered experiences, hardships, aspirations, and strengths of those with PNES. The volunteers in this book have shared in such a vivid and representative manner that which I have heard over the years and which now, through this book, will be available for all to read, and they have exhibited profound bravery in sharing with the world what it is like to have PNES. I suspect some may have agreed to participate in this project to help others who are part of the PNES community (the newly diagnosed as well as the ones who have been dealing for months or even years). By reading this book, others with PNES may learn that they are not alone and, in fact, are part of a community with a voice. Others may have agreed to participate in this project to communicate with the health professional community in hopes of being seen as human beings deserving of care and respect.

I am optimistic that this Brainstorms volume will produce a significant and positive change in the lives of those living with PNES (patients and caregivers) and in how many of our colleagues in the field of health will perceive this group of patients in the future, with all their nuances and complexities. The voices on the pages that follow are loud and clear, and if we take the time to hear them, they have much to teach us.

Lorna Myers, PhD
Director, Psychogenic Non-epileptic Seizures Program
Northeast Regional Epilepsy Group, NY, USA

FOREWORD

Amanda Payne

I feel honored and proud to contribute this foreword to *In Our Words*. For so long, those of us who have been diagnosed with non-epileptic seizures have felt unheard and alone. Now our voices have been gathered together, and our stories are here for everyone to read.

This book is the result of a collaboration between medical experts and people diagnosed with non-epileptic seizures, also known as non-epileptic attack disorder (NEAD) or psychogenic non-epileptic seizures (PNES), depending on where in the world you live. No definitive statistics of prevalence currently exist, but in the United Kingdom (UK), a country of sixty-five million people, a similar number are estimated to have NEAD as have multiple sclerosis—somewhere over a hundred thousand people. Those diagnosed suffer a range of symptoms, the main one being seizures that look like epilepsy but that are not caused by the same abnormal electrical activity in the brain. Everyone is different, and their seizures can vary from those resembling tonic-clonic style attacks to absence-type seizures in which the person just stares blankly to unusual actions such as walking in circles or shouting and more. Currently, getting diagnosed correctly takes an average of five years. People are often initially misdiagnosed with epilepsy and may end up taking unnecessary medication for several years.

One of the biggest difficulties is that the condition is so little known. Despite a big increase in research and awareness during the past few years, many general practitioners, Emergency Department doctors, and the like do not know about it or understand it. This can sadly lead to a person being accused of attention seeking or "faking" at one end of the spectrum or being seriously overtreated and medicated at the other. A book like this should go a long way to help both those diagnosed with NEAD and those trying to help them to have a better understanding of what it is really like to live with this condition.

What struck me most about the stories in this book, written by people from all over the world, is the strength of the people telling them. Their lives have been turned upside down. They have lost their independence, their jobs, and in some cases, their relationships, yet they are still willing to speak out and share what has happened to them so that others might gain strength from their experiences.

There are many emotions laid out here: disbelief, sadness, and anger (especially anger), but also hope. We hear not just the people who have the seizures but also those who love and care for them. Some can clearly define what set the cycle of seizures into motion (e.g., a traumatic event, abuse, or an accident); others are unable to find a cause. Historically, these types of seizures were considered to be purely psychological in origin, but it is increasingly clear that a physiological element is involved as well. Research is beginning to show links with migraines, with sleep disorders, and with chronic pain.

People describe their seizures in different ways. Some people have an aura, a warning of what is coming, while others have no warning at all. Nearly everyone describes how terrified they were the first few times that it happened. It is hard to put into words exactly what it is like – that feeling of losing control over your body.

Some of the stories are hard to read. People describe the struggles they have been through to get a diagnosis and treatment. Some describe how they have been treated in hospitals, at work, and even by their own families. There is a lot of emotional pain laid out in black and white on the page.

As I said earlier, however, there is also hope. Getting the diagnosis can be a big help, especially if it is given in the right way by a specialist who knows what he or she is talking about. A lot more information is available now, with more research being done and more specialist clinics opening. Online communities are bringing people together to share their stories, and to relate what worked for them and what didn't. Treatment options are available that weren't offered before. There is still a long way to go, but we are definitely starting to see a light at the end of the tunnel.

My own story is very similar to the ones in this book. I was treated for epilepsy for five years before getting the correct diagnosis. Then I was given a sheet of paper with a website address on it and told there was nothing more that could be done. At the time, there was very little information or support available, and that prompted me to do something. I started a group on Facebook, which grew and grew. With the help of specialists, I created a website for NEAD. Two years ago, I joined forces with some other people, and we formed FND Action (http://www.fndaction.org.uk), a charity for those diagnosed with functional neurological disorder, of which NEAD is one. FND Action has just passed its first birthday, and we are working hard to raise awareness and provide support and information to those diagnosed.

What helped me more than anything was talking to other people with the same condition. Understanding that I was not alone—and that I wasn't crazy—made an enormous difference. My hope is that this book will help others like me. I'm so grateful to everyone who contributed their stories and to the editors for gathering them together. I hope that you, the reader, gets as much out of this book as I did.

Amanda Payne
Director of FND Action, a UK–based Charity
for those Diagnosed with FND (Functional Neurological Disorder)
and NEAD (Non-Epileptic Attack Disorder)
Chatham, Kent, UK

PREFACE

Previous books in the Brainstorms series have demonstrated how much readers (both lay and professional) can learn from those whose lives have been affected by epilepsy. Having initially given a voice to individuals around the world who experience epileptic seizures themselves, and to their families, subsequent books in the series provided a forum for health care professionals to share their personal experiences of epilepsy and help close the gaps that sometimes exist between health care users and providers. These books have made a huge difference to readers, many of whom have subsequently shared their own stories with the senior editor.

The current volume is the first book in the Brainstorms series that does not focus on epilepsy. Non-epileptic seizures go by many different names (including psychogenic non-epileptic seizures, non-epileptic attack disorder, dissociative seizures, conversion seizures, functional seizures, and pseudoseizures). All of these labels describe episodes that can look very similar to epileptic seizures but have a different cause and are experienced quite differently. People with epilepsy typically perceive their seizures as something external to them, a hostile or threatening enemy that acts independently of their own will and does something to them (e.g., causing them to move involuntarily, rising up inside them, or knocking them over). By contrast, non-epileptic seizures are more commonly experienced as a state people go into or a place they get transported to that is not normal and in which they may feel stuck.

Unlike epilepsy, which is caused by abnormal electrical activity in the brain, non-epileptic seizures are an involuntary response to triggers inside or outside the body that the brain perceives as threatening in some way. Triggers inside the body include physical sensations (e.g., pain or fatigue), emotions (e.g., fear, anger, or frustration), and certain thoughts or memories. Triggers outside the body may be particular situations that people find themselves in or things that they see, hear, or smell. These triggers do not actually need to be dangerous or threatening—they only need to be perceived as such by the individual on some level. For instance, a person's brain may link a particular smell with a sense of danger because this smell was present during a threatening situation in the past. Importantly, the brain may respond to triggers very quickly. Seizure triggers may therefore never have had time to actually enter the person's awareness, which could explain why non-epileptic seizures often seem to happen "out of the blue." Once the brain makes these connections, it may then cause behaviors such as those described in this book.

In many ways, the mechanisms causing non-epileptic seizures are similar to those that can lead to panic attacks. However, whereas in a panic attack the triggers for the episode cause fear, loss of control, an impending doom or dread, or a sense that one may be about to die, the triggers in non-epileptic seizures cause an automatic response that can be compared to what happens when a computer "freezes." When this has happened, the brain will only function normally again once it has "rebooted." And when the brain is working again, the seizure will have helped to move the individual from the brief moment in which the brain detected a situation that could be a threat to a state in which the seizure may have left the person confused, embarrassed, exhausted, upset, tired, or achy, but where the initial perception of threat has gone away. In this sense, non-epileptic seizures may serve a useful or protective function by allowing the individual to escape the situation, perhaps even with less distress than they would have experienced in a panic attack.

Although quite a bit of medical evidence for this explanation of non-epileptic seizures exists, the processes in the brain that cause these seizures cannot currently be visualized by any test or examination. Unlike in epilepsy, where the epileptic activity causing the seizure manifestations can show up in electroencephalographic (EEG) recordings, no currently available test can demonstrate the changes in the brain that are responsible for causing non-epileptic seizures. Of course, this does not mean that non-epileptic seizures are not real, or that individuals are making up what they are experiencing. Indeed, countless other conditions do not produce any changes in the brain that can be visualized by routine tests—for example, migraine headaches, and many other disorders characterized by involuntary abnormal movements. However, the fact that the processes leading to the development of non-epileptic seizures cannot easily be seen or measured objectively means this diagnosis is commonly overlooked and delayed by several years.

The road to being diagnosed with non-epileptic seizures is often long and winding. Non-epileptic seizures tend to feel like a "physical" problem to the individuals experiencing them, although doctors usually think of them as a "psychological" problem. Most people who are eventually diagnosed with non-epileptic seizures are initially given the incorrect diagnosis of epilepsy and prescribed anti-epileptic medication. Often, the first clinicians who individuals see regarding their non-epileptic seizures are not seizure experts, and given the difficulties in diagnosing this condition, doctors consulted subsequently may disagree with the initial assessment or with each other. Sometimes the diagnosis can be even more challenging, as about one in ten people with non-epileptic seizures have additional epileptic seizures. Other people may have had epilepsy in the past, and then gone on to develop non-epileptic seizures. Even when a correct diagnosis of non-epileptic seizures has been made, individuals are often given a short or poor explanation by their doctor and sent away with no further support, unsure what the condition actually is. Not surprisingly, they may find it difficult to accept or understand the diagnosis. This is especially un-helpful, as it is hard for people to get better without understanding the nature of their condition. Although some specialist services for individuals with non-epileptic seizures exist, these are not available everywhere, and access may be limited even where they are.

Many publications in scientific journals and books elaborate upon the medical understanding of non-epileptic seizures. However, it is much harder, especially for those having non-epileptic seizures themselves, to find out about the experiences of others without medical jargon. We have therefore created this book as an almost unique resource providing insights into how non-epileptic seizures affect people's lives. It contains stories of despair, frustration, adversity, and raw anger, but also accounts of challenges faced and overcome. Many of the writers in this book criti-cize how health care professionals have responded to non-epileptic seizures (espe-cially those involved in providing emergency care), but others describe individual clinicians who managed to make a very real and positive difference in their lives. This is often achieved by simply listening, taking the person with non-epileptic seizures seriously, and answering their questions. Ultimately, most people with non-epileptic seizures manage to find a way forward, which means that the seizures become less disruptive and disabling. In these accounts, "patients" become their own healers.

The original meaning of the word *patient* is "the one who suffers." Those with non-epileptic seizures suffer from their attacks, experience anxiety about the next seizure, worry about the effects of their seizures when inside and outside their home, and encounter isolation and stigma resulting from their condition. They also en-dure treatment in emergency departments, long waits for neurology appointments and tests, confusion about insufficient or inadequate explanations, anger about the lack of access to treatment, and disappointment and apprehension about therapies that may not work. Much of this is not unique to those who experience non-epi-leptic seizures. These are the sorts of things that many other "patients" have to put up with as well, including those with epilepsy.

However, in this book, the contributors stop being "patients" and turn into people who take action. Even the writers of stories describing a passive endur-ance of their suffering are asserting themselves by sharing their experiences. And through telling their personal stories, they are showing others with non-epileptic seizures that they are not alone. Although there are as many different stories in this book as there are authors, there are also some experiences that many of the writers share with each other (and perhaps with the readers as well). This should go some way to reassuring those with non-epileptic seizures that they are not going crazy, and that their experiences are common and very real.

In addition to speaking to others with the condition, the stories in this book will help to inform professionals providing social, educational, or med-ical services to individuals with non-epileptic seizures about what it is like to live with this problem. No paramedic, nurse, or doctor who has read these accounts is likely again to think of non-epileptic seizures as something people could simply stop doing at will, something they could easily control if they just tried a little harder, or something they are doing just for attention.

Last but not least, by telling their stories, the contributors to this book place a responsibility on those organizing health and social care to develop adequate services for people with non-epileptic seizures. Current approaches to non-epileptic seizures are reminiscent of how people with epileptic seizures were discriminated against in previous centuries, before the medical profession recognized the biological basis of epilepsy. The individuals who have helped to fill the pages of this book with their experiences are not content to continue suffering in silence. Combined, their voices form a powerful chorus: There is no reason why non-epileptic seizure disorders should not be treated at least as well as epilepsy or any other condition that is thought to be "fully explained" by a narrow biomedical view of disease. There is no justification for discriminating against people because the seizures causing their distress and disability are not associated with epileptic discharges in EEG recordings.

The process of collecting and reading contributions to this book has been a deeply humbling and illuminating experience for the editors. We are endlessly grateful to the writers, who have shared their personal thoughts and experiences with us, and to you, the readers of this book. By contributing to this book, the authors have done more to move forward the understanding of non-epileptic seizures than any scientific treatise by the editors (or other professional experts) could have done. The generosity, dignity, and courage of the authors have earned our deepest respect.

We invite all readers who would like to share their own stories or reactions to this book to write to contact@fndaction.org.uk.

Markus Reuber, Gregg Rawlings, and Steven C. Schachter

ACKNOWLEDGMENTS

We are grateful to everybody who has contributed to this book. The following contributors are acknowledged in alphabetical order; the remaining authors wished to be anonymous.

Steven Ackroyd
Trudy Angus
Kate Anscomb
Charlene Atkinson
Linda Baer
Carolyn Barker
Gail Barry
Beverley Beckstein
Danielle Birrell
Jayne Bishop
Aleta Burgess
Bryony Carleton
Tracy Cawley
Celia Cherry
Ed Cole
Victoria Jane Cole
Carmen Coleman
Dennis M. Daniel
Stephanie Douglas
Diane Dunsmuir
Laura Edmonds
Nicola Edmonds
Ellese Elliott
Mark Ericksson
Tammy Evans
Alison Farrant
Barry Gordon
Haley N. Gordon

Joanne Gordon
Joanne Molloy Graham
Annemarie Grant
Tiffany Greer
Sarah-Leigh Hardwick
Rachel Hay
Stephanie Hodgson
Hannah Holden
Jason Hopfauf
Michael Hrehor
Carol Anne Jackson
Graham Jackson
Richard Wentworth Johnson
Eveline de Jong
Mandy Joyce
Sandra W. Kanyoro
Jumana Katar
Zoe Lancashire
Andrea Leach
Francis Louis LeClaire
Lisa LeClaire
Kay Lindsay
Margaret Anne Carol Livesey
Deborah Lomax
Kathryn Longbottom
Patricia Longbottom
Pamela R. Loughlin
Charley Maidment

Sarah Mason

Alison McCready

Judy Mielke

David Napier

Eric Nelson

Bridget Noonan

Sharon Ooley

Lorraine Otsmane-Elhaou

Tanya Palmer

Lisa-Marie Patrick

Charlee Pearson

Wendy Pickering

Marjolein Praet

Ceri Pritchard

Lisa Richardson

Sharon Ross

Veronica Santiago

Arthur van der Schaaf

Sharla Seeds

Tony Short

Dustin Simmonds

Jennifer Simmonds

David L. Spangler III

Jasmine Streatfield

Rebekah Louise Sutherland

Kate Taylor

Amy Treslove

Simon Wadsley

Charlotte Ward

Vicky Warriner

Sarah Wenger

Lindsey Woodward

We thank the following organizations for their support in helping make this book possible:

Epilepsy Action

Epilepsy Research UK

Epilepsy Scotland

Epilepsy Society

FND Action

FND Hope

Medical Humanities Sheffield, The University of Sheffield

Neurology Psychotherapy Team at Sheffield Teaching Hospitals

(NHS Foundation Trust)

Nonepilepticattackdisorder.org

Northeast Regional Epilepsy Group

And we also thank the following people:

Dr. Hamada Hamid Altalib, Yale School of Medicine, USA

Dr. Ian Brown, The University of Sheffield, UK

Professor David K. Chen, Baylor College of Medicine

Associate Professor William Curt Phillip LaFrance,

Jr. Brown University Medical School, USA

Dr. Lorna Myers, Northeast Regional Epilepsy Group, USA

Dr. Dilraj Sokhi, Aga Khan University Hospital, Kenya

Dr. Hasan H. Sonmezturk, Vanderbilt University Medical Center, USA

Professor Brendan Stone, The University of Sheffield, UK

Ms. Joanne Huckstepp, Sheffield, UK

LIST OF COMMON ABBREVIATIONS

CT   Computerized Tomography
EEG   Electroencephalogram
MRI   Magnetic Resonance Imaging
NEAD   Non-Epileptic Attack Disorder
NES   Non-Epileptic Seizures
NHS   National Health Service
PNES   Psychogenic Non-Epileptic Seizures
UK   United Kingdom
USA   United States of America

COVER ARTWORK

The cover artwork is by Joanne Huckstepp. The piece is entitled "Torn":
"I have begun to understand how and why I became so ill
I couldn't have prevented it, I'm not super-human and I'm not to blame.
Therapy has made me stronger and has given me the confidence to process what's
right and what's wrong for me as an individual.
I can now make the changes to enhance my life—I just need to paste my broken
self together again."

1

Person with Epilepsy and PNES, UK

My way of describing non-epileptic seizures is that I stare into space, mumbling, looking very pale and with heavy eyes.

I don't have many friends as they think I am strange due to the moves and noises I may make. I don't go out around town etc. as I can't drink pints and waste money on smoking so I don't mix in. I do some odd things when I come around like dusting, sweeping up, washing up, or walking around in circles.

My family has always been able to explain to other folks and shops what my trouble is after breakages etc. in supermarkets. My mind is blank; I can speak then stop in silence until it is up.

I have had many different jobs, one for thirty-six years. Firm sold up, new job, new contract, different firm, but due to my seizures, blackouts, and rules of health and safety, I was thrown out of the job for my own safety and the safety of others working with me, moving machinery, fork trucks. I am unemployed due to the health and safety officers because of my seizures and my age. No one wants to know about employing me to cover their backsides due to any accidents happening to others or me. I can't work with machinery, can't climb, and can't drive.

I have had some part-time jobs since, but my age and seizures go against me now, and computer-wise I am very thick, can't look at screen for long as it seems to affect me.

I don't seem to have any confidence in myself.

I never had girlfriends up until I was at work with the lass who come to my aid when I collapsed on the floor. We married. She was deaf and dumb at one time; we have two children, boy and girl, plus one grandson and one granddaughter.

2

Person with PNES, UK

There is no, nor has there ever been, a standard seizure; however, all of my seizures have been characterized by a sense of loss or diminishment of one's usual sense of control over oneself, an experience of impaired agency. Typical phenomenal features include a rushing sensation, like your blood is hot, a spasm of energy that contorts the muscles. It is like a foreign body has taken control and there is an internal tussle for power. You are no longer in the driving seat; there is some argumentative lover in the front with you, trying to grab the steering wheel. It is like being drugged, and the trip is usually negative. It is as if you took an ecstasy pill at church, or the supermarket—it just ain't the right time to be gurning at God or twitching out on the dance floor at the local supermarket. All the while your cognitive abilities are still intact, somewhat observing all this internal/external kafuffle, sometimes bemused while other times fearful. The psychiatric evaluation afterwards injects a bit of trauma into the mix, as this is the apparent etiology of such phenomena, so you're now sitting uncomfortably in your physical and metaphysical chair.

Sensations include a numbing or prickling around the lips and especially the eyes, which feel compelled to roll down the back of your head. A deep sleeping sensation can suddenly wave over, causing random snoring, a complete sense of inertia or feeling as though you are walking through water. Everything becomes heavier, like the opposite of floating on the moon, sinking into the ground so much so one would just lay motionless on the surface of the earth, contented albeit. This is also accompanied by a flat affect, yet the physical symptoms of emotions seem to remain, like the heart racing or slowing, the muscles contracting, etc. A state of sudden trance and the body compelled to dance to some terrible, inaudible techno music. And just a general irritability because of the adrenaline. It can make you pretty arsey and cold, very cold apparently—I am told like a psychopath. It's not pleasant in this aspect, and without feeling the mind strays too far, beyond the borders of morality, as there is nothing holding it back except a memory that you are a good person. Yes . . . I hope.

Day-to-day life used to be quite different when they first began eight years ago. Back then I was quite embarrassed, I had no idea what was happening, I thought I had epilepsy or a tumor. Physically they were quite inconvenient and drew attention when it was not desired. I found it difficult to perform the simplest task. It was not so much the impairment itself but more so the disability; that is, the social barriers that come with this condition I found were huge. However, this isn't the seizures as such; this is seizures in the context of society. The seizures would be quite tiring; I would feel afterward that I needed to sleep. Sleep was like a reset button; even if I weren't tired, I would try and sleep. It would be quite difficult to remember what was going on around me, and generally I felt quite "out of it."

Now I feel that they come when I experience emotions intensely. If I feel very happy, I may get a pain at the back of my head and begin to twitch and feel light-headed; then the happiness seems to fade away, so intense emotions, other than anger, are few and far between. Anger seems to be the most frequent emotion, and it's not long before I am angrily twitching. Likewise, if I try not to physically express my emotions, the seizures are all the worse. Physical contact with my lover can be difficult, and so can an emotional connection. This greatly affects our relationship as I always appear to be distant, or saying that I do not want to be touched in a certain way as it might set them off.

My family members at first didn't believe me, and accused me of faking seizures, which was very hurtful and I think was a blow to my pride (I was always proud), especially to sink as low as to feign a serious illness for attention, as I thought I was too important to stoop as low. So it baffled me indeed that they would jump to such conclusions. My mother, I must say, at the time was the worst. My friends also were mean to me during the seizures. I was aware of this as I could still hear. Work colleagues appeared concerned, and eventually my employer said that I was unable to continue to work for him due to the disorder. My doctor laughed at me while I was experiencing an episode as my face contorted and I stuttered though the conversation. The paramedics assaulted me as they said they didn't believe that I was having a seizure. My therapist would only partially listen to my story, and I must say that he had the most extreme case of cognitive bias—not a scientific man at all.

The condition was first explained to me terribly. I was diagnosed by a neurologist with a purely "psychological" disease, nothing to do with the brain, and given a pamphlet. I cried in the toilet of the hospital for an hour at my unexpected diagnosis of madness.

I had cognitive behavioral therapy for two years. I can't say if it helped or not. I think the act of speaking can itself be a relief. However, the conflation of bad memories with good when told to envision my happy place, and then remember being raped, tarnished the best memory I had. Pretty unforgivable.

When I first received my diagnosis, I was confused; now I realize it's they who are confused.

Certain things have helped me cope with my seizures. To not forget the power of forgetting and truly moving on with my life. Trying to create a controlled and peaceful environment seems a catch-22 as I get so stressed about trying not to be stressed. I cry when I can, shout, run, moan, and laugh, but sometimes I can exert myself enough and the surge trips my circuits. I think the most terrible act about this whole saga was being diagnosed with such a contrived mythical disease. The way I got over this was to study the philosophy of mental disorder and realize that indeed, as Aristotle thought, men will create diseases, in name at least, so that they may sit in their ivory towers, or their comfy recliner office chairs. I'm sure there are some who believe that they are doing an honest day's work, but so do some policemen.

3

Person with PNES, Australia

During 2011 and 2012, I started having very severe upper body seizures. This would result in my body being propelled backward at speed and anything I was carrying would go flying—you should see the roof in my lounge where the television controller has hit it. These were up to six times a day at one point, then five to six times a week. Eventually, through my own ability to better control the spasms, things started to get better. I am not allowed to walk outside for fear of seizures or falling, and I still must have a carer with me at all times; my beloved wife usually fulfills that demanding role.

The seizures are a constant reminder that I have to take it easy, I have to stay safe and not put myself at risk, and outside I have to be in my wheelchair at all times. A timely warning of this happened the other day as I was sitting in the pub having lunch when I had a seizure. It was so violent that it thrust me backward, I overbalanced in my wheelchair, my knees hit the table, and I was saved from serious injury by my wife grabbing hold of my chair. Very frightening.

4

Person with PNES, Canada

The first pseudoseizure that I can remember woke me up one night at camp where I was a staff member in the summer of 2007. I found myself shaking; when it stopped, I felt exhausted. Once I gathered enough energy, I got up and told the other camp counselor in our wagon (it was an Old West–themed camp). Neither of us were sure what to do, so I went back to sleep. In the morning, I mentioned to the camp director that I thought I might have had a seizure, but they didn't seem too concerned since I hadn't had seizures before. Someone wondered if the hot weather might have been a trigger. It was several years before I had another episode, and I didn't think too much about it.

I believe that my first symptoms of conversion disorder occurred between Grades 8 and 9. I had a close call involving lightning. It blew out the phone that was a few feet from my head. At the time, I thought I had been hit; now I doubt it since I didn't actually feel anything, nor were there any signs of electrical burns. Whatever happened, I was quite ill in the following weeks. I had one more menstrual cycle and then they stopped (to this day, if I am not on birth control to regulate my cycles, I get one cycle once to twice a year). My muscles ached for weeks after, and I was so nauseous that I struggled to eat, causing my weight to drop from 135 to 114 pounds.

About a month ago, I suffered a pseudoseizure while on my bike. Fortunately, I felt it coming, so I was able to stop before it fully hit. It was about 5:30 p.m. on Friday night on my way home from school. I have about an hour bus ride between the university and the mall; I sometimes take my bike to get around the campus. Someone saw me (actually I ended up stopping directly in front of him) and got me off my bike. Some kids who were in their yard got their father who called paramedics. It was a cold day, and the ground was damp so they got me some blankets. When the paramedics arrived, they got me into the ambulance pretty quickly and then started asking questions. Apparently, the paramedic supervisor was nearby, so he arrived on scene about the same time. So I had three paramedics asking questions; in the meantime, I kept having more episodes. I found it pretty overwhelming.

I generally tense up and shake (at least that's what I feel like I'm doing, it usually isn't very obvious to people around me except for my immediate family). When I am having an episode, depending on the severity, I may or may not be able to respond, but I've always been totally aware of what is going on.

The decision was made to take me to the hospital. The paramedics had never heard of conversion disorder/functional neurological disorder but were quite understanding. I was taken directly into acute care on arrival at the hospital. The paramedics stayed with me for about an hour until a bed was ready. I gave as much background information as I could, but my memory was a bit poor at the time, so details on which medications I'm on were a bit difficult to remember until we/ I located my purse and found the one I couldn't remember. One of my warning symptoms is that I become foggy, and thinking/memory becomes difficult. I may feel a bit shaky. I continued to have episodes on-and-off during the evening. A bit later, I had a bad episode where I began shaking quite violently. Another nurse saw me and started talking to me to get me to respond for a few minutes. "What's wrong? I need you to tell me." I couldn't respond, so she asked another nurse if she knew what was wrong with me. When she was told pseudoseizures, she left. I don't like being left alone when they are happening. It was probably about twenty minutes until I felt like I would have been able to respond to anyone or move. For the first part, I was shaking, and whimpering a bit, then depending on the severity, I typically feel very tired and drained when it is done. The emergency doctor came by a few minutes later. I gave him the story as best as I could. I called them pseudoseizures. He asked why I called them that. I said it was what I had always been told they are. I know what happens. He said that's what it sounded like. He ordered my thyroid blood levels, tested to make sure that they hadn't gone way out of whack, and hurried on to the next patient. Then a head trauma patient came in. Sometime around that point is when my dad got there. I may be breathing pretty hard following an episode trying to shake the tired and drained feeling. My nurse helped me get to the washroom. By this point, I was pretty weak, and still having shaking and spasms. The rest of the evening we spent waiting for the results. Once they came back, I was sent home and told to see my psychiatrist, who had just left on vacation. It was about midnight by the time I was released that evening. So my on-campus general practitioner monitored me for the first two weeks. Then I saw the psychiatrist when he got back.

I discovered the morning after that I had missed my Friday morning medication, which may have been a factor. And because it was so late when I got back, I mistakenly took my morning medications at bedtime, so I had a poor sleep. On Saturday I was not in very good shape; I was really weepy, tired, and weak. To get some rest, I made the decision to spend several days at a place that offers community housing for people with mental illness. I took several days off of classes to rest. I was pretty weak after. I should add that I've had two periods of three months where I was having difficulty walking to the point that I've had to use a walker. I was starting to struggle somewhat with walking again after that evening, so I have been working with physiotherapy before that could worsen.

Since that weekend, I have been having several minor episodes on most days. I usually go really tense each day; my back and neck sometimes arch back, generally lasting about ten seconds or less. Sometimes it will go on for a few minutes. It is rare for people around me to notice that anything is wrong unless I am directly in front of them. Usually my mother is the best at noticing my symptoms. My dad often doesn't notice.

It is interesting to note how dogs respond to these episodes. If it is an episode where I am really convulsing, my dog will start barking, which gets my family's attention. If I'm on the floor but not shaking, my dogs will come lie down with me until I can get up. I've been able to train my dog to help me off the floor, or stabilize me on stairs.

I've been at a friend's house, and their dog noticed that I was having trouble before anyone else did (I don't remember exactly what the dog did, but I think she came and tried to nuzzle me).

5

Person with PNES, USA

I had my first series of seizures in 2013. These lasted over the course of a week and then subsided. I was seizure free until the spring of 2015, when I was hospitalized for a seizure that lasted four hours. I have been having seizures regularly for the past nine months. I have not yet been seizure free for a month. My seizures often do not seem to have a trigger. At first, I thought that they were stress-related; however, they happen just as often when I'm calm.

My seizures are usually five to ten minutes in duration. Prior to having a seizure, I have an aura. My auras can last anywhere from five minutes before the attack to a few hours. My auras are very uncomfortable and often involve the contraction of my abdomen muscles as well as pain in my side and upper back. Because my seizures involve dissociation, I usually experience a fight-or-flight sensation just before a sei-zure. I feel as if my body is in overload, and I often panic. The panic is heightened if I am in a place with a lot of people or if I'm unable to get somewhere private. My seizures usually have two parts—a period of violent convulsions and then a period of numbness right after. After my first convulsion, my body feels a tingling feeling that can be attributed to the dissociation. From that point on, I am unable to speak or control my limbs. I cannot hold thoughts, and my mind feels completely blank. I feel as if I'm separated from my body. Although I am not all the way "there" during my seizures, I can still hear everything and am aware of what is happening. My abdomen, legs, and arms violently convulse. I often hit, kick, and punch the ground and/or objects in my path. I sometimes also make moaning and choking noises. After the convulsions stop, I feel very disconnected to my body. I describe it as feeling "dead." I am unable to move, and my face/body is stiff. This lasts for approximately three minutes directly following the convulsions. After I come out of my dissociative state, I feel as if I'm just waking up in the morning, yawning and stretching my muscles. On occasion, I regain full cognitive and verbal functioning, but I am unable to feel portions of my body. This kind of partial paralysis can last up to thirty minutes.

I do not like to have anyone in the room when I'm having a seizure. If I'm not at home, I will often go into the bathroom to avoid someone seeing me have an episode. My seizures can be very traumatic for me, and my worst feeling is that someone else has to feel the panic that I do. I find that when people do see me have one, they do not know what to do. They try to talk to me, which makes things worse. I am a teacher. When I first started having them at school, I found that the staff panicked.

My seizures make me feel isolated. After an event, I find that I want to talk about them to the people I'm close with. While my close friends and family are good listeners, I find that they do not know what to say. I feel like I am a ticking bomb waiting to go off, and I feel like people are scared to be around me because I never know how long I have before I lose control. I try very hard to control them, and sometimes I can drag the aura process out for a substantial amount of time; however, I become very discouraged when I still have a seizure despite my efforts. The longer I try to control my body, the worse the aura gets until it is simply unbearable. I start to stumble, lose fine motor function, the room gets blurry, and my breathing gets heavier. My seizures also make me feel hopeless. I have gone up to three weeks without having a seizure. When I am seizure free, I feel motivated to fight because I feel like I've won and maybe they won't come back. Unfortunately, they always do. When I have bad days, I feel defeated. It's hard to fight when you feel like you've done everything to stop them but they just won't let up. Since I was formally diagnosed, I've felt more frustrated and anxiety-ridden about my seizures. I want to get better, but because the research is so lacking, I have trouble believing that I actually will. The thought of "having to learn to live with it" scares me and has made it difficult to concentrate on anything else. Even on good days, my body is exhausted. Activities that I used to enjoy, such as taking walks or going to the mall, require a nap afterward. I'm moody because I have no energy and my body feels weak. This condition has affected my ability to hang out with my friends and has made going places by myself difficult.

I currently work fifty-plus hours over the course of a five-day workweek. I love my job and have worked very hard to establish my career. My seizures happen at work. So far, I have been able to avoid having seizures in front of colleagues; however, I fear that one day it will be inevitable. The disabilities coordinator for our county is watching me closely, which makes me worried that I'm going to lose my job. Focusing on your needs and listening to your body at work is difficult when you are worried that someone might find you incapable because of your disorder.

I've seen countless doctors over the past few months. I am angry about the way I've been treated by them. I have a history of an anxiety disorder that I have worked through years of therapy to manage. When I go to the doctor, this seems to be all that they see. They dismiss me and attribute my seizures to a psychiatric condition. At this point, no one has explained treatment options. Doctors send me home with nothing but the diagnosis. In fact, most of my understanding of my illness has come from my own research. I feel that doctors aren't willing to go the extra mile to assist me with managing my disorder. I've repeatedly presented them with patterns along with research; however, they do not want to acknowledge my ideas.

At this point, nothing helps all of the time. I find that food plays a role in the frequency of my attacks. I switched to a gluten-free, soy-free, and dairy-free diet about six months ago, and I am finding that my disorder is more manageable. Since then, I have experimented on occasion with introducing these ingredients back into my body. Sometimes I am okay, but sometimes I am not. My seizures are much worse when I am ovulating. I find that if I eat these foods during that week, I am prone to episodes. Recently, I have also found that exercise can be helpful. I try to push myself to exercise at least five minutes per day, although my body is exhausted.

6

Mother Whose Daughter Has PNES, UK

The purpose of these few paragraphs is to describe our experience as a family living with our daughter who experiences non-epileptic seizures. My daughter is now fourteen, and the attacks started two years ago, the December after she started high school. Her first episode was at home in the middle of the night when she collapsed in the bathroom, hitting her head against the wall. We didn't have a clue what had happened. That was the beginning.

The seizures have varied over the last two years, both in frequency and length. My daughter tends to fall to the ground with little warning and can "black out" for over an hour and twenty minutes. She can sometimes get a headache before and after and feel very tired afterward. The fall happens quickly, and occasionally, she has hurt herself. Many attacks started to happen at parties and school. At school, she could fall downstairs, and without a diagnosis, they would call an ambulance in case of injury and she would end up at the Accident and Emergency Department for hours on end. Sometimes it would look like she couldn't breathe properly, which would scare people a lot; other times she just looked asleep. She is totally "out" and doesn't respond to anything mainly.

When I think about why she is having them, looking back, my daughter has always shown a degree of anxiousness in certain situations—I remember when she started primary school that she would always have a tummy ache and did not want to go in, or didn't want to go to dance classes or join in at parties in front of people. Starting high school has been a challenge for her; this big change seemed to start the episodes the December after she started high school. Other triggers seem to be hormones and heat. We realized getting a diagnosis was very key to dealing with the episodes and people around us. I think that my daughter becomes overwhelmed with "worries," and when she is totally overloaded, she shuts down.

Regarding experiences with medical professionals, initially both general practitioners and consultants just told us it was her age and that she would grow out of them. But with six seizures a day and being "out" for over an hour sometimes, we pushed and pushed to get a proper diagnosis/referral. Ambulance staff were sometimes very supportive, but I remember one paramedic indicating that my daughter was putting it on and she should just snap out of it, which was really frustrating. My family and I started to do our own research and came across non-epileptic seizures; I could tell from the description it was highly likely that my daughter had this condition. I then had the confidence to challenge health professionals and skeptics and to try and avoid her being taken to hospital. I do remember there was hardly any support while waiting for a diagnosis, well none that was forthcoming anyhow. Luckily, I work at a hospital, and so I popped into the Neurology Department after seeing a banner detailing non-epileptic seizures and after doing some internet research. They were amazingly helpful after the man at the main reception desk told me how he had a friend whose son had just been diagnosed. He gave me advice, and I took it. He also asked a consultant to speak to me, and she was really helpful. They signposted me where to get help and how to get a diagnosis and reassured me that we were doing all that we could as a family. The school nurses had no idea about the condition; the medical room has been fantastic, but they also had little experience at the beginning. They are now experts . . . mainly because there is another girl in my daughter's year who also has the condition and her mum is a teacher at the school. Strangely, they seemed to trigger each other's episodes as well, having the same condition. The school made many adaptations to ensure that they could deal with two girls experiencing together twelve attacks or more per day.

Having received a diagnosis has helped my daughter cope. She has now been taught coping strategies from her psychologist. She hasn't accepted that there isn't an underlying medical condition causing them, which we need her to do to move forward. The episodes have now decreased from six times a day to a maximum of twice per week. She uses relaxation and has apps on her iPad, which I know she uses. We also talk to her more about situations/stresses/worries and how to deal with them. Social media plays a part I am sure! My husband and myself are also working closely with the psychologist and school, so we are all on the same page. She has avoided certain situations, which she knows can cause her attacks, such as large crowds.

Thinking about family and friend's reactions, some have been really great and supportive and read articles to understand the condition. However, one family member did surprise me just recently when she said my daughter will be better when she isn't looking for attention, indicating that she was doing all of this for attention. I soon put her right. Local friends have been brilliant when episodes have happened. Her school friends become a little medical team and understand what to do during an attack, recovery position, etc. Parents have helped in situations when attacks have happened, ensuring her safety. Attacks have happened by roads and on stairs at the cinema. We ensured that parents had our mobile numbers and tried to ensure that my daughter still leads a normal life, but I do find myself getting very anxious when she is out and about. Some of my daughter's "friends" have drifted away or said some quite hurtful things as they felt like she was holding them back, particularly as attacks happened on school trips or days out with friends and parties. There are examples of adults even talking about how she is doing this all for attention; this is the minority, but very frustrating.

Regarding examples of attacks and the implications, my daughter was enrolled on a watersports school trip this year, but the school told us in the end that she couldn't go as we were still waiting for a diagnosis. I was actually relieved, but she was devastated. Many attacks happened on stairs at school—every time the phone went off when the seizures were at six per day I was extremely anxious, scared about the implications of falling. For now they have reorganized lessons so that she doesn't go upstairs at school anymore. I still get very nervous when she has a bath; logically, it is no longer likely to happen in our home but . . . what if, so I always ask her to leave the door unlocked and stay upstairs. My husband is a bit more relaxed than me, and so it has caused us to have many "discussions" over certain boundaries. This has got easier with the diagnosis and support. She has missed a lot of schooling due to seizures, and we are trying to work with her and the school to manage this. My work has been very supportive, and when the seizures were at their worst, they ensured I had time off to deal with things. We also had to put our two-year-old into full-time nursery care to ensure that we could manage what was happening. This of course then had a financial impact on the family. I remember my daughter having an attack at a concert at the local arena. It happened right where many thousands of people were trying to exit the concert. Luckily and coincidentally, one of the stewards came to help, and his wife had the same condition. We managed to avoid an ambulance by explaining the condition to the medical room there.

There are a few things that could have helped more:

1. The information available while waiting for a diagnosis is very limited. Some websites were extremely helpful for us, but local services had no idea about the condition, including school nurses/medical room staff/local general practitioners. More awareness is needed.
2. Paramedics and school nurses should be trained to understand the condition as it isn't rare!
3. Support while waiting for diagnosis—to me, this is a crucial stage where you need help/advice and support as a family. I had to search for this myself.
4. General practitioners need to understand the condition more. There is limited information out there about pediatric non-epileptic seizures.
5. The waiting time to see a specialist is so long! The process was really challenging. I eventually gave up and tried the private route to speed things up, and even this was difficult.
6. From talking about this to other people, I have found that there are many others out there who are going through the same thing. A support group for carers would be really helpful, or even a link to people going through the same.

To sum up, we now feel like we are in a totally different place after the diagnosis. The hardest part is definitely getting the diagnosis, and then when you know what you are dealing with, it becomes easier. My daughter is getting much better, but we still need her to accept the condition and what it is. Her episodes have decreased from six per day to a maximum of two per week. She sees a psychologist for one hour per week, which has played a huge part in this decrease of episodes. I do worry what happens when these sessions come to an end; I worry about them increasing again.

This is written from a carer's perspective—for my daughter, I know this has caused her great distress at a time when she is wanting to push boundaries. She has felt embarrassed at certain situations, tearful, frustrated, and confused. I admire how she has coped, and it has made her stronger and has made her realize true friendship. She just wants to be treated the same as anyone else. I am very grateful for all the support we have had over the last two years. We have a long way to go, but we are definitely getting there.

7

Person with PNES, USA

I had my first seizure at work in February of 2012. While at work, I started staring off into space; a coworker came over to ask me a question, and I was unable to respond. I could hear and see him, but I was not able to respond. I heard him calling out that there was something wrong with me and to call 911 [the emergency number for the US]. In my head, I was saying, "No, I'm ok." I can remember thinking that I should talk to him—he's calling 911. I finally spoke, but when I did, I stuttered out the words. That was my first trip to the hospital in an ambulance. I was perfectly fine when I reached the hospital. They said that I was just simply dehydrated and released me.

Now and again for the next few months, I started to feel strange. My equilibrium was off. I felt lightheaded, and I had headaches all the time. I would stare off into space. I had had symptoms like these in the past and had seen a neurologist, so I decided to go back to him. He could tell that I was in bad shape, but when he took an MRI everything was normal. He wasn't sure what was wrong, but he started to treat me with medication. This medication, however, made my headaches worse. I had a headache every day, and he just kept telling me to take more pills. I was up to five pills a day (I later found out that this is normal until your body gets adjusted to the drug; he never told me that). When I went back to him, he suggested a sleep apnea study. I wanted no part of this because everyone I knew was being tested and they all strangely seemed to have it. It seemed like a scam to me. He was also, I thought, very condescending to me because I tried to explain to him that it was more of a sharp pain in my head that would come and go, and not like the constant pain of a headache. I never went back to see him. (I do regret this because I believe he was trying to help.)

My next seizure happened at work. Again, I was sent to the hospital, and again, I was fine. I was only a little dazed. That is when the doctor told me it must have been because of the migraines I'd been having, although she also told my sister and me that sometimes people faked seizures for attention. Of course, she didn't believe that I was doing that! She then suggested I see a neurologist.

When I went to the neurologist, he laughed at what the Emergency Room doctor told me. Migraines don't cause seizures. It was my heart. So I wore a heart monitor for three days. Nothing turned up on the monitor.

Once a doctor was able to witness my seizure, he said that it wasn't a real seizure, it was a non-epileptic seizure, and he gave me another form of medication. He also told me to see a psychiatrist, and I was stunned. He never told me why he gave me this form of medication. I believe it was because he also thought that I might have fibromyalgia.

When I felt the next seizure coming on, I had a friend drive me to the Emergency Room. After waiting for six hours with a splitting headache, I had a seizure in the waiting room. With my eyes rolling in back of my head, my arms flopping around, and my head shaking swiftly back and forth, they finally decided to take me back. I received another MRI and a CT scan, and they hooked up my brain to electrodes to view my seizures. They came back with non-epileptic seizures again. I went back to the neurologist. I liked this doctor. He explained to me what non-epileptic seizures were and what they thought caused them. The problem with that was that I hadn't been sexually abused or physically abused; I hadn't been treated by a psychiatrist except when I lost a child twenty-five years ago. I was stressed, but who wouldn't be? I left the office numb. The doctor asked if I could have been abused and blocked it out. For the next year, I kept having more and more severe seizures and trying to remember if I could have been abused. Every time I went to my primary care doctor, he would bring up if I had been abused. He even cornered my ex-husband, asking him questions about whether I was abused. I was still having a hard time dealing with my diagnosis. I didn't fit the norm for these seizures.

I continued to have seizures, but my doctor wrote a note with instructions, and my coworkers stopped calling 911 every time I had one. This was a big relief because the stress of all the hospital bills wasn't helping my seizures.

My next seizure lasted twenty-eight minutes. I was completely out of it. My eyes were glassy and rolled back in my head; I wasn't able to complete sentences and was talking gibberish. Everyone in the room was crying (I was told), and when the paramedics arrived, one of my coworkers told one of the paramedics that I had seizures and asked him to take me to the hospital where my doctor was, but he refused. As the other paramedics got me on the cart, he came up to me and hit me hard in the middle of the chest. I cried "Ouch!" He told the other paramedics I wasn't having a seizure. I heard them whispering that they thought it looked like a seizure. By this time, I was coming out of the seizure, and I was livid and asked again to go to my hospital, but he still refused. We argued about which hospital to take me to. I knew I had to go to the hospital because I still didn't feel right. Once we got to the hospital, he proceeded to tell the nurse that I was faking. I then witnessed the nurse mouthing to the doctor and other nurses that I was faking. I had enough, so I refused to stay at the hospital and signed my discharge papers.

A few days later, I contacted the hospital to report the nurse. I was told that she would be reprimanded and made to do a report on non-epileptic seizures. I also reported the paramedic; however, he denied that he had hit me, and for some reason, it never made it into their report.

After this, I decided that I needed to know once and for all what exactly was wrong with me. I went to a hospital that has a specialist epilepsy unit. My doctor encouraged me to go, hoping that I would then be able to accept my diagnosis. I was unimpressed with this hospital. I spent most of my time in the waiting room waiting for them to fit me in for tests. They did the same tests that my doctor did. They too found a V-shaped artery in my brain, but were not concerned, because it did not appear to be an aneurysm. Once again, I was diagnosed with non-epileptic seizures. I guess I had to accept it now. I went back to the doctor to let him know that I was ready to accept the diagnosis, only to be told that no one in my city dealt with non-epileptic seizures. He could recommend a psychiatrist, but they didn't specialize in non-epileptic seizures.

I was discouraged, but I called the number only to find out that there was a six-week waiting list and my insurance wouldn't pay for it. I found someone on my own only for her to harp on to me about my weight and send me back to the neurologist. "Nothing wrong here!" I decided to just wing it; all the literature I read said that very few doctors knew about psychogenic non-epileptic seizures.

I continued going to work every day until the seizures got worse and I had to quit. My son was going off to college in another state. He insisted that I come with him. For about a month or so, I had very few seizures. Then they returned with a vengeance, and I couldn't always predict when I would get one. I have stopped driving. I still try to joke about them, but it is harder for me to go out. I don't want to embarrass anyone. At this point, my seizures are pretty violent. I fall to the floor, and my head shakes violently from side to side. (Sometimes my neck hurts for days afterward). My feet and legs shake, usually knocking off my shoes, and my eyes roll back in my head. Sometimes even the littlest of things will set it off, like lights, noises, and even telephone ringtones. Sometimes I think that my eyes play a factor, but every time I go to the eye doctor and they shine the light in my eyes, I have a seizure and they immediately stop the exam.

My family wants me to go on disability, but I'm fighting it. I haven't worked in a year. The worst part is that sometimes I feel like I wish I had cancer or some other typical disease. At least they would know how to treat me. I wouldn't be in limbo. Most of what I know I learned on my own from the internet. I've learned things like stress could be a factor. Most importantly, I learned not to give up. So, I will call another psychiatrist, only to be told that they can't help me unless I know what's causing the seizures. I will continue to email people, especially people on television, to help promote the awareness of this condition. We need for this to be a priority. We are sick, just like people with a heart or lung disease. We need help and right now, but there is none. There is shame in our disease, but it isn't our shame! It's the medical professions' shame. "DO NO

HARM," well it's too late for that. The harm has already been done by the way the medical professions have treated us. Although there are as many patients with non-epileptic seizures as there are with multiple sclerosis, very few studies are being done for non-epileptic seizures. I keep telling myself it could be worse; they locked people with epilepsy up in psychiatric wards for years before they realized what was truly going on. I guess we'll just have to wait until the medical world catches up!

8

Person with Epilepsy and PNES, UK

When I first got the diagnosis, I didn't feel relieved at all; I felt like a freak. My family was supportive, and at that time, my husband was too. After a number of failed attempts to find the right medication and dosage, I eventually did, and I'm seizure free. Is this the time to say yay and end the story? Ha, it is hell. That was just the beginning.

In my early twenties, epilepsy had yet to make its appearance. The non-epileptic seizures were slight and few, and I was able to ignore or find excuses for them. I could drive, and had a full-time job with progression and prospects.

In my thirties, I had a series of tonic-clonic seizures. It took eighteen months to get a diagnosis of temporal lobe epilepsy. I was told that all my other symptoms were linked to the epilepsy. It took a further two or three years at least to get on a medication that worked and that I could stand the side effects of. None of these medications affected what I was feeling except for the tonic-clonic seizures. I was reduced to part-time work.

In my forties, epilepsy was no longer a problem, well-controlled with medication—but other symptoms were becoming worse all the time. Unsympathetic employer providing no support. Could no longer drive. Began falling a lot. I had to leave my job. No benefits available to me. Not able to walk far without support, so no independence. Confidence zero. Relationship with my husband fast going down the pan. Finally, after years of questioning doctors, I received a diagnosis of non-epileptic seizures.

The future—who knows.

Having a diagnosis that makes sense is a huge relief. My husband is trying to understand and support me, and has at least stopped mentioning the D word (divorce), so we may get through this. Hopefully, in time, I can reclaim some of my life. I don't think I'll ever be quite who I was before, though.

My family just accepted my diagnosis of epilepsy without fuss. Whether because they didn't know much about it or would just accept me whatever I had, I don't know, maybe a bit of both. Questions started when I didn't seem to get much better over the years and I had no answers to give. Finally, after years of emotional upset, and trying various doctors, consultants, neurologists, and whoever else for answers, not to mention countless tests and scans—it would fill a book on its own to go into details—I finally got a diagnosis of non-epileptic seizures as well as the epilepsy. I had worked my way up the medical profession to seeing a professor by this time!

Family didn't really understand what this was but accepted it all the same. My sister's comment of "you're brilliant, just do what you can do" was the most touching and became my mantra for a while.

If only my husband's response to it all had been so straightforward. Then again, he was in the middle of it, day after day. When I first had epileptic seizures, I think we both thought that all my symptoms were epilepsy, I would start taking tablets, and hey, presto, I would be fine again. He held on to this idea long after I had abandoned it. It took him a long time to come to terms with the fact it was going to be more complicated than that. He found it hard to see me having seizures long after the tonic-clonic seizures were sorted out. We were told for years that these were part of the epilepsy, and as you do, we believed what the doctors told us.

Over the years, I got worse and worse, I was able to do less and less, and my life got smaller and smaller. I lost the ability to drive, my independence, confidence, job, financial stability, and all the things that we used to do as a couple went because of this. No more day trips, meals out, holidays, country walks, and countless other things. Due to either my physical failings or financial instability, I, now we, lost it all. I had enough just trying to cope with each day. No wonder he was fed up with what our life had become; I was too.

Things had to reach a climax. I had got to the point where I could not even walk far without needing someone to hold on to. I had fallen so many times, always backward, hitting my head on the ground. We knew the way to the Accident and Emergency Department very well! Injuries suffered in short order—fractured skull, broken wrist, lacerations to the back of my head, concussion, vertigo, loss of sense of smell, cracked ribs, and many, many grazes and bruises, not to mention loss of my self-esteem! And all the while neurologists etc. were being quite happy to let me leave their offices despite the fact that I kept on falling and despite the fact that none of them seemed to be able to find a feasible reason to explain it.

Then a few things happened at once. My husband saw me fall more often and couldn't stand to see it or deal with the aftermath. We started to talk about separating; although neither of us really wanted to, we couldn't see another way out, any light at the end of the tunnel, or any future where we could be happy. And lastly, I was referred to a professor where I finally got a diagnosis of non-epileptic seizures.

None of us really knew what this diagnosis meant, and we had to do a lot of trawling around for information. In the end, though, we decided we could now try to improve how things had been, both medically and emotionally.

My husband found it easier to support me, armed with a bit more information, and I no longer had to hide symptoms and falls from him because I had thought it would be another nail in our relationship coffin. Now I knew it wouldn't be, he wouldn't get mad, and we could work through whatever came up.

Slowly, I am trying to reclaim my life, with his help and support. We have started going for short walks again. We may have to walk arm in arm and slowly for a bit of it and stop if I have a "wobble," but we are doing it. Hopefully, I will get a bit better over time, and other things will follow. I don't know what the outcome will be, but I feel more positive about the future now than I have for a long time. I may only be able to do half of the things that I used to, but I would not have even been able to achieve that without the understanding and support of someone I love and trust.

I suppose the moral of the story is that you can't do everything alone, sometimes you need someone to understand what you are going through, trust them to do their best to support you, and be able to talk things through with them no matter how personal or daft it is or sounds. Without that person, I could not see any future where I could be happy, be "able," keep my marriage alive, or indeed have any future worth having. Now there is at least a crack of light at the end of that long dark tunnel.

9

Person with PNES, UK

This week, I am going to see my doctor. My appointment is at 10 a.m. on Wednesday; therefore, we need to travel to the hospital on Tuesday as it is out of our area. I am very apprehensive about, firstly, the journey as it is such a long way from home and, secondly, the appointment.

Journey: Last time we travelled any distance was in July for a family holiday with our daughter, son-in-law, and two granddaughters. The holiday had been planned last year when I felt as though I could cope with life a little better, but December came and everything health-wise seemed to deteriorate faster than the previous two years. However, our journey to the hospital went without a hitch; we stayed in a local hotel for the night, and things ran relatively smoothly. My appointment with the doctor was fine, although I was very apprehensive due to the fact that over the last three years I have had such a negative reaction from medical professionals regarding my illness. I don't remember much about the journey, but in my case, that is not unusual as my brain seems to react to stressful situations by blacking things out. This wasn't helped by our daughter, who seems to have been in denial of this illness and unable to discuss things with me. I have struggled a great deal with this as in the past we have been able to speak about anything and everything; however, in the previous week, there was no contact from her regarding my appointment and I desperately needed her backup but, as always, my dear husband was there by my side and, as always, gave me all the support he could.

The appointment with the doctor was very relaxed and extremely enlightening. It was wonderful for me to speak to someone who understood perfectly what I was going through and to give us some positive advice; both my husband and myself felt much relief after we had seen him as we now know what we are dealing with.

10

Person with PNES, USA

Before I was diagnosed with non-epileptic seizures, most nights I awoke with that worms-crawling-in-my-legs feeling, and many nights I awoke with my right leg and arm thrashing about the bed. My head twisted to the left, and I was afraid I might not be able to breathe. When it stopped, I got out of bed and paced the floor for the rest of the night, worrying. I was terrified, and even more terrified when it happened to me at work or other places at the oddest of times. I recall that someone had laughed and said that I had gone over the rainbow and was tap dancing there. It wasn't funny then, and the remembrance isn't funny now.

After several attacks of whatever was happening, my closest friends from work brought me to the Emergency Room, where I was poorly treated. I was admitted and given enough medication that I totally blacked out for five days; I recall absolutely nothing.

While I was in the hospital, I underwent both an MRI and a CT scan. Both tests appeared normal, but I appeared anything but.

Then the diagnosis was made; it stated that I was having pseudoseizures and that I was crying out for help. I was wide awake when I heard those words.

My entire body dropped, and I emotionally wrapped my arms around myself. I agree; I was crying out for help. I was begging for relief from my pain. I was pleading to know what was wrong with me. I implored their aid to put an end to these seizures. Fear, like a wound, opened up inside my spirit.

Another time, I had seventeen seizures, one after the other in a single night. My head was screaming in pain. I went to the hospital only to have the Emergency Room doctor get inches from my face and say, "Ohh, you have a headache? Do you want a pain killer, or is it a narcotic pain killer you're looking for?!" What an ass! Know that he was reported. Seizures and needing help in the Emergency Room don't say that we are addicted to opioids! Don't take the baloney, ever!

The seizures continued. Many! I had to be weaned from the anti-anxiety medication. The withdrawal from that medication alone was complete hell! I suffered depression deep enough to nearly drown in a well of pain.

I was out of work on medical leave for five months. I was a manager in a health care center. I lost my job. I did return to work, but in a lower capacity. It really is okay. I am doing what I love, being with residents who love me and accept me right where I am.

My body, mind, and spirit continued to cry out, but this time for loving support.

A neuropsychologist with whom I spent an entire day evaluated me. Just months ago, I was evaluated once again. Everything appeared okay, but there was a recommendation to have another MRI or CT scan in the right frontal area of my brain. I chose not to opt for that. The others before that showed a minimally damaged portion of the mathematics area of my brain. It's in the frontal area. So . . . I have trouble with mathematics. Calculators help a lot!

I saw and still see my therapist regularly. I also saw my psychiatrist and continue to seek her care regularly. I feel accepted and respected. They have witnessed my seizures firsthand. I take medication daily for these seizures. The medicine I take is an anti-epileptic drug. It does help. However, I do have seizures occasionally.

It was when I was poking around on the internet to try and find some information that would provide details about the seizures that I finally found the answer. I stumbled upon a site where I felt welcome.

As I read, I learned that seizures such as mine that did not appear to be epilepsy were called psychogenic non-epileptic seizures, also known as PNES. To finally have an appropriate name for my condition both exhilarated and relieved me!

What I am sure of is that this condition is treatable. While I continue to have seizures, I know that I am not crazy and that I will be okay. However, while giving the seizures the name PNES helped me immensely, my reaction to every seizure then and every seizure since is . . . I HATE THEM!

My seizures come in clusters. They are all on my right side. I can tell one is coming with the tiniest twitch in my right fingers and wrist, and have just long enough to say, "I'm going to have a seizure now!" Lately, though, I've been surprised to find myself in the throes of the seizures before I can account for it. I usually have three seizures—one, then a minute later another, then another. Those seizures can last a minute or more. An hour or so later, I have what I call a "big" one that is more severe and lasts longer. I cry. I swear. My right leg burns and spasms at the end of the seizure. My right arm burns as well, and then becomes very cold.

Post-seizure I am exhausted, nauseated, and my balance is off. This can last and usually does for up to five hours. If I am in a place where I can rest, I try to lie down for at least 30 minutes. At work, they are understanding and provide a place for me. When I am out and about—say, on the street—it's a different story. Yikes! I have been fortunate to have someone who knows me or a kind person to bring me home. I don't drive. Also, after seizures, I have balance issues—I tend to lean to the right for up to two weeks at times. I may have trouble finding words or say the wrong words. Sometimes I just cannot think. People have a bit of a time understanding my post-seizure issues.

My seizures have occurred in some interesting, shall I say, places. I am always upset wherever and whenever I have a seizure, but in these places, oh my, I was mortified! Once on the altar in church. Another on a plane just as we were heading down the tarmac! Thank goodness I had time to tell the man sitting next to me about my seizures. My wrist began a telltale twitch that told me I'd better talk fast. My daughter was there to help him and me. The people across the aisle watched. At first, the woman thought I was afraid of flying, then understood I was having a seizure. She waited for me as I departed the plane to make sure I was okay. What a sweet woman!

I hate the shaking. I hate the jerking, bending, and twisting. I hate the crying. I hate the swearing. I hate the burning pain and the spasms.

I have a special person in my life who gives me love, support, encouragement, and who cares about me enough to be honest with me when I need that as well. I am surrounded by the acceptance and love from my friends and family.

There's something comforting, though, when people with any condition come together with others who share the same issues.

Being healthy encompasses all our parts, not just our physical body. When our emotions are in turmoil or our mind is bombarded with obsessive thoughts, our health is compromised; we already know the result—seizures. It is important to create balance in our lives by nurturing our entire selves. It is paramount to our total health to meet our spiritual, mental, emotional, and physical needs.

If we feel balanced, we will experience joy in what we do. We will have a sense of purpose and feel that our lives have meaning. We will treat ourselves with love and respect. We will also be loving and respectful with our loved ones. We will feel calm and less stressed and anxious. That can lead to a quieting of our seizures.

I write. Poems and short stories come through inspiration from my brain, which still works quite well, despite the seizures. The writings help me get through the bad and enjoy the good times.

I think the biggest help I have given myself to try and quell the seizures is to let them go. Truly, it isn't easy, especially when they can occur so often. But by saying to myself "Breathe and let them go," they're over. Let's get on with the good part of life. I truly believe my seizures have lessened. What occurred weekly, sometimes more often, with the help of medication, yes, have now become every two to three months. I am grateful for that. I wear a bracelet, a pretty one that has the word "breathe" on it. I look at it daily. I have to remember in uncomfortable situations, and before, during, and after seizures, to breathe. It is a precious piece of jewelry to me.

Now . . .

Together, we say as a community of friends:

PNES . . . finally it has a name!

We are comforted and comfortable.

We feel acceptance.

We are not alone.

It is not the end.

Be blessed with healing in your body, mind, and spirit.

May your seizures be quieted.

THE LADY WHO WAITED

Once upon a time, there was a lady who waited. She didn't want to tell them that she was in pain, and shaking, and crying, and swearing, and burning yet again.

So, she waited.

She couldn't wait much longer, the pain, and shaking, and crying, and swearing, and burning was making her see stars and feel sick. So, she called the doctor and waited on the phone.

The receptionist told her that there was a wait for an appointment, so she should wait at home, by the phone, until someone called her.

The lady hung up the phone and waited.

The nurse called and told the lady to wait a little longer while she told the doctor. The lady continued to wait. While she waited, she felt dizzy and nauseous, and the pain, and shaking, and crying, and swearing, and burning kept coming, and those stars kept coming when she tried to move her head. But, she waited anyhow.

After a wait, the nurse called back and said, "The doctor said that you need urgent care. Don't wait any longer. Go right to the Emergency Room." The lady didn't wait and did what the doctor ordered. The lady met a very nice receptionist and two very nice volunteers at the Emergency Room. They saw her when she had pain, and shaking, and crying, and swearing, and burning. They were kind to her while she waited. And waited. And waited some more.

A nurse came out and called her name. The lady went into the examining area and waited a bit. The nurse came in and wrote down what the lady said. Then the nurse took the lady's vital signs and told the lady to get undressed and wait for the doctor. The lady felt dizzy and sick while she waited, and waited. And guess what, once again the lady had pain, and shaking, and crying, and swearing, and burning. And once more she saw stars and felt sick.

Just then, the doctor came in. He asked the lady what she wanted him to do. The lady said, "Please find out what is wrong with me when I have pain, and shaking, and crying, and swearing, and burning. I am afraid. I see stars, get dizzy, and feel very sick." The doctor looked in the lady's eyes. He made her touch her nose, look up there and over there, stand up, close her eyes, and stick out her tongue. She felt like he was giving her a sobriety test. He did not ask about her pain, and shaking, and crying, and swearing, and burning. She waited, thinking that he might do that.

The doctor told her to wait and a nurse would come and take some blood. The nurse did come and take some blood.

And the waiting began again. Waiting. Waiting. Waiting. It seemed like a very long time that this lady was waiting. The doctor returned and said, "I really don't know what you want. You can go home now. If in a few days you are not better, call your primary physician." The doctor said that the nurse would come and discharge her. He left the Emergency Room cubicle. The lady began to wait. The lady dressed and waited, and waited, and waited.

Finally, the nurse came in and spoke kindly to the lady. The nurse was a kind nurse. This time, a different nurse, a man. But, he had to tell the lady to wait. Finally, he got the papers to discharge her. He gave them to the lady, touched her shoulder, smiled, and said, "Good luck. I hope you feel better soon." The lady wanted to cry.

The lady went home to wait and see what would happen to the pain, and shaking, and crying, and swearing, and burning that was making her see stars and feel sick.

What do you think happened?

Yup, she still has the pain, and shaking, and crying, and swearing, and burning that makes her see stars and feel sick. Waiting for the pain to get better. Waiting for things to change.

She is still waiting.

11

Person Who Is Now Free of Epilepsy and PNES, Canada

I had epilepsy as a child. It was terrifying and set me apart from other children. Due to my seizures, I had to relearn how to do everything; as a nine-month-old, I was a newborn in everything but age. My seizures also gave me a learning disability called auditory processing disorder. I know that you want to know about my experience with non-epileptic seizures as an adult, but it is impossible in my mind to speak of one and not the other.

As a child, I only ever got a seizure when accompanied by a fever. To this day, I get nervous when I get a fever, even though I know that my body will not have another grand mal seizure ever again. As I grew up, brain plasticity worked in my favor. It has never been fully explained to me as an adult, but I remember being told that my brain changed so much that it would be medically impossible to have another grand mal seizure. (Looking back as an adult, I doubt the words *medically impossible* were said, but that is how I remember it.)

Maybe my nerves stem from a learned behavior as a child. That is not really important to you, though. My greatest fear as a teenager was my seizures coming back. I remember how the kids never looked at me the same after I had a seizure at school, how adults got scared every time I got the flu, how not remembering the thing that everyone was scared of made it that much scarier, and how I have never felt so free as the day I was told that I did not have to take any more medication for my seizures.

The last time I took medication for my grand mal seizures, I was in Grade 4, maybe 5. Fast forward to some point in my mid-twenties, I have never had had a great memory, but I started to notice more and more people were telling me we had had conversations and done things together that I had no recollection of. This scared me as the last time this happened was as a child after a seizure—I would tend to lose about a week's worth of memories. I was certain, though, that if I had fallen on the ground shaking and peed myself as an adult, someone would have at the very least told me, or a more likely scenario, I would wake up confused in the hospital like I used to. So, since no one noticed anything, naturally I was being paranoid. What else was I to think? I thought surely this is my teenage fear acting out on me as an adult. So I carried on living and was just confused by conversations and things that I apparently had done but had no recollection of.

Time goes on and I start developing this severe abdominal pain. I thought my appendix had burst, it hurt so much, but the pain was in the wrong spot. My abdomen always hurt, but it got to the point where I was going to the hospital at least once a month and the doctors just kept telling me I was okay. During these events, I often didn't know my age, and once I even forgot my name, but that was written off as I was in so much pain that I couldn't focus. I underwent so many blood tests, ultrasounds, and scans and tried many different medications to help figure out what the problem was. Nothing was showing up; every doctor at the hospital just kept telling me I was okay. My general practitioner believed me, though; he seemed as determined as me to figure out what the problem was. They even went down my throat and up my bum with scopes to try to see if there was something not showing up on the scans. Once again, though, nothing that explained my pain. My sister-in-law mentioned that she happened to be watching a television show about a doctor who makes difficult diagnoses and heard about something called abdominal seizures. As all this was going on, the pain was so bad that I was on bed rest. I have never felt so alone, hopeless, and dirty as when I was stuck in bed. Sure, I had my family and my boyfriend, but they were able to leave. I was stuck. Since I never went anywhere and was unable to take care of myself, I had people looking after my needs. People would carry me to the washroom and put me on the toilet, then leave the bathroom, and then help me to the sink afterward so I could wash my hands. Then back to bed. This went on for a year. In that time, though, people were watching me more than they ever had to before. They started to notice that there were times I was staring off into the middle of nowhere, and apparently I did something with my face that was unusual. This led me to have a diagnosis of complex partial seizures. I thought, "Oh, shit! My worst fear has come true," and at the same time, "Oh, thank God! A diagnosis that means there is hope out of this mess."

My "complex partial seizures" were even scarier than my childhood seizures. I could be sitting in a room with people, and it was as if my brain pressed a pause button on life, then suddenly, with no warning, people would seem to be teleported to another part of the room or miraculously appeared without any warning. The scariest of these was when my husband was in the kitchen, then suddenly he was sitting next to me with his arm around me. My diagnosis, however, did not give me a way out of the mess that I had found myself in. My seizures became more and more frequent, even though the medication was supposed to be helping to get rid of them. I had the same terror as a child, and I had time taken away from me again.

I am not sure of the timeline of things. I know things were bad and then got a bit better for a year (I went and did a condensed year of college to receive a diploma in professional counseling). I received my diploma in early September and got married in November. Then my memory all but disappears from my first year of marriage; I remember my wedding day, my honeymoon, and that is all the good memories I have. A few months after being married to the love of my life, and my best friend, I lost my memory in a horrific way. I basically woke up one day and couldn't remember my life. From accounts of people in my life, I would ask for a glass of water, and in the time that they would go and get me one, I would have forgotten that I had asked for it. By the time they came to give me my glass, I would look at them so thankful and say, "How did you know I was thirsty? Thanks!"

There are two events that I remember from this year that I wish I could forget. The first was during a family reunion that happens in the same place every year since I was a little girl. I was out sitting on the cabin's porch, and I looked around at all my family there and wondered where grandpa was. Then like a wave I remembered he had died years ago. I left the porch quickly and went to the basement, where I had to grieve the loss of my dear grandpa again and alone. No one would understand how I had forgotten that grandpa died, and I did not want to have to explain myself. I don't know what hurt most, having to deal with the grief while my family was happy around me or having to deal with the fact that I had forgotten that grandpa had died. Even writing this down is causing tears to leak from my eyes and feeling the pain as if it was happening yet again to me. When you only have two memories from a year of your life, it can be too easy to relive them over and over again.

The second memory is much less painful but confusing. At the time, my husband and I lived in my parents' basement suite, and I woke up early one morning (which is unlike me) and was confused as to why my brother's room looked so odd and why I was not sleeping in my bed. At this point, my brain didn't even have a clue that my husband was asleep next to me. To make things more complicated, my childhood bedroom pretty much looked the same. I went upstairs and curled up in my bed and fell back asleep. In my mind, I knew with every core of my being that I was sixteen. Then I thought my husband would miss me, so I came downstairs. That is the power of love; no matter when in time I jumped, I always knew who my husband was, even though at sixteen I did not even know he existed yet.

Since I have no memory of this year, I do not know the events that took me to the seizure clinic, but I found myself in the hospital with wires attached to my head, being videotaped for everything, but going to the washroom while a nurse had to stand at the door. I was there for nine days. Every time after I thought I had a seizure, I pressed a button so they could look at the tape and the readings from the EEG. I felt depressed and scrutinized. On the ninth day there, I was told that I had non-epileptic seizures. They showed me the results over the last nine days. At first, I did not believe the test results. It seems not only improbable but also impossible.

I went home full of despair that the medical system seemed to have failed me yet again. Over a year of being told that I was okay by doctors when I was in severe pain seemed like a bit much. I suffered for about another six months, and then I contacted the psychiatrist that talked to me during my stay at the hospital.

I thought that even if I thought she was wrong, at least she seemed to think she was right and had an answer for me. No one else did, so I thought that as a last-ditch effort, I would go see her. Best decision of my life.

Through my treatment for neurological functional disorder with my fabulous psychiatrist, I am now seizure free. I went back to school to be a legal administrative assistant, and I am currently working in my field as just that. If you told me even three years ago that this is where I would be today, I would not have believed you as I was unable to drive, remember things, or take care of myself. As horrible, de-pressed, and hopeless as my life used to feel, I now feel terrific, joyful, and hopeful. The journey to my recovery was long and I am not done yet, but it's nice to feel like a functional human being once again.

12

Partner of Person Who Is Now Free
of Epilepsy and PNES, Canada

So my story about my wife and her seizures starts not that long ago. We met in 2004 and started dating at the end of 2008. Then, in October 2009, I finished my shift at work and turned on my phone to find a message that she was in the hospital. When I got there, I was told that she was having severe abdominal pain. Having just had my gall bladder removed, I figured we were looking at something like that, but it was not to be the case. Shortly after I arrived, doctors informed us that all the tests that they had run came back as negative, so they gave her some painkillers and sent us all on our way.

Thus began the initial saga of my wife's first bout of bed rest, and the monthly hospital trips, and trying different hospitals to see if someone could give us an answer. Those months were incredibly difficult. It's impossible to describe how it feels to see one of the strongest people you know unable to do anything without assistance. I also noticed that she was having significant gaps in her memory, which wasn't too alarming at first because she has never been a person with a great memory to begin with.

Eventually, we met up with a neurologist who thought she might be having abdominal seizures, and who prescribed anti-seizure medication, which seemed to clear things up enough that she went back to school for a year. Other than a brief episode during a really stressful practical test for her course, life seemed back to normal.

It wasn't until a few months into our marriage, around February 2012, when I got another phone call. I was told that my wife had collapsed in the kitchen and had "lost" about four hours of time. When I say lost, I mean that she had no recollection of time passing or what she was doing in that time. This began another series of regular visits to the hospitals, and to specialists, who seemed stumped as to why this would be happening and why the medication would have stopped working.

It was also during this time that her memory began slipping away from her more and more. She would forget asking me to grab something for her in the time it took me to retrieve whatever she had asked for and return with it. I started leaving her notes in the morning when I went to work so that she didn't panic when I wasn't home and would have some idea of when I'd be back. I watched her disappear, a little piece at a time, helpless to do anything but try and give her some small comforts. I'd see her appear to zone out and lose all concept of what was going on around her.

About a year and a half later, still with no answers, we found ourselves at the seizure clinic. Through some of the observations I and others had made, we were initially given a diagnosis of complex partial seizures, which we were told would explain the episodes where my wife would "zone out" but not have any other visible seizure activity. While the episodes were still occurring, it was somewhat of a relief to be able to give a name to what was going on. Shortly after, my wife was booked into the hospital to remain under observation so that they could record any seizure activity.

They did not find any. Instead, through a psychiatrist working at the hospital, it was determined that she has a functional neurological disorder, where her body can manifest stress as physical symptoms, in her case the seizures and memory loss. As luck would have it, this psychiatrist specializes in this disorder, so my wife has really had some great care and is now able to live a normal life, albeit with medication.

I would be lying if I said there wasn't a part of me that was worried something could trigger this again. But it's nice to know that she has a solid support system and we have some ideas as to what to do in the future.

13

Person with PNES, UK

Around August 2008, my body started to become off-balanced—I would find myself unable to walk straight, and I started tripping up over nothing. About the same time, I really hurt the muscles in my lower back. My husband had injured his back at work, and moving to a new home had agitated it, so he was laid up and I was having to go do the shopping, and walking back home pulling shopping trolleys is how I hurt my back and is when I noticed my balance being off. This went on until December 2008, when things got worse, as I started falling to the left (never right).

On the morning that I had booked an appointment with my doctor, I had a strange turn. I fell backward onto a chair; my husband said that I looked deadly white and disoriented. My first thought was that I had a transient ischemic attack (strokes/heart attacks are in my family), and I was on cholesterol medication. We attended the doctor's appointment, and she did tests (I had a definite weakness in my left leg). She sent me off with a letter to a Medical Assessment Unit near to the hospital. I remember having to walk into town to get some money for the bus. I really did not feel like it at all. The bus ride was twenty minutes, and then we had to change buses to get to hospital. I was really tired and drained. I got sent for a chest x-ray. The doctors debated whether to send me for an MRI but eventually did. Not sure in hindsight if that was a good thing! During the scan, I had my first ever seizure. I had walked into the unit but now could not stand or stop violently shaking—even the wheelchair was shaking and I was feeling very scared. We still had to wait to see a doctor; I remember one was really nice, but the other was adamant that this was just a reaction to some new anti-depressant medication that I had been given. My husband kept telling him that I had not started those yet as I was still in the weaning-off period of the other medication.

I was given this diagnosis of non-epileptic attack disorder in 2010 by a consultant. I felt bewildered, angry, confused, but at least he said the symptoms were real. I did my own research but found contradicting information—I got told to ignore the violent shakes, recite something in my head while trying to walk on jelly legs, breathe slowly in through my nose and out through my mouth. I cannot seem to regulate my breathing while having a violent attack, and so I hyperventilate; the fact that I am asthmatic does not help.

They say once you accept your diagnosis that it will get easier; this was untrue for me. I am constantly looking for answers—why, what is wrong with me, can I get help, is there a cure, will it go away as quickly as it started. I also ask myself why is it that some medical professionals don't believe my condition is real.

Over time, I have had cognitive behavioral therapy, seen a psychologist and a psychiatrist, and had physiotherapy on my legs. I take antidepressants and muscle relaxants.

But like all conditions, proper research takes years and money, and I think that the world is only just beginning to take this condition seriously. My understanding now is that I get a malfunction between my central nervous system and my brain; somewhere, the signals get distorted.

I have lived with this problem for eight years. We (my husband and I) have learned how best to cope with my symptoms; we have learned to adapt to accommodate non-epileptic attack disorder. For us, the only way is forward.

14

Person with PNES, UK

Let's start before my first episode. My health is generally good, although low back pain has been a limiting factor in most of my adult years. Oh, over the last 15 years, I have had many surgical operations, including four on my spine, cataract removal—both eyes—and follow-up laser treatment are the most recent procedures. My working life ended in redundancy [in the UK, redundancy is a form of dismissal from your job] in 2002, and removal of a vertebral disk in my neck happened a couple of weeks after. My work in the computer industry, plus redundancy, plus that major surgery add up to considerable stress. I coped with it all. My mental health has never been an issue—it's likely that a diagnosis of Asperger's syndrome would be made if I were a child now, but I cope with being awkward in social circumstances. ("I ain't bovvered" comes to mind!)

Now fast forward to August 2, 2014. When reaching up high to remove a television wall bracket from the top of a cupboard in my garage, I lost control of its arm, which swung around and hit the side of my nose. Dazed, but probably with no loss of consciousness, I went indoors to my wife and recovered. However, I felt groggy most of the time and saw my general practitioner six days later: concussion. About two weeks later, I had an "episode" in which I slumped and could not respond to my wife's worried questioning. During this episode, I was scared, then I began to regain control, and was very relieved to find that I could move both feet/hands/ cheeks etc. In other words, this was not a repeat of the transient ischaemic attack a couple of years previous. After four such "episodes," I saw my general practitioner again . . . and again and again. Now, about one hundred episodes later, consultations with two neurologists, visits to the psychiatrists at the elderly persons' mental health services, x-rays, and CT scans.

I had three "episodes" on Christmas Day with my home full of family members showing their concern, support, and love for me. I feel fortunate to have them ... and fortunate that incontinence hasn't been a feature of any episodes. My seizures do affect what I can do, but I'm coping with that. My focus is to manage the attacks as well as I can. I accept that they may be psychogenic, but I'm not yet convinced that there is no physical link. Too many attacks have been triggered by a blow to my head, including the latest one last Monday.

15

Person with PNES, UK

Being diagnosed with non-epileptic attack disorder was both good and bad. It was good in the way that it allowed me to put a diagnosis (or tag) on my condition, but bad as it seems socially misunderstood. It seems people think you are either making it up or that it isn't a real condition/diagnosis. My parents and myself struggle to understand that it is mainly a psychological disorder as I am normal and don't have any mental health issues. In fact, the diagnosis makes me feel like I am mental, almost like they are putting words into my mouth. It is almost like they can't find a reason for my unconscious episodes and can't be bothered to investigate properly, so they've just whacked the stress label on. My dad suffers from anxiety and depression, so I can't discuss it with him as it makes him feel like I've inherited his bad parts, which makes him worse (he tries to hide it from me). My mum finds it hard enough dealing with my dad, let alone me. My boyfriend is amazing and always says we will find a way to deal with it. My friends dismiss it.

I am a nurse, and I have worked on a neuroscience ward. We have a patient whose mum has pseudoseizures, and the nurses always mock her or say she is weird and fakes seizures—these are professionals and even they don't understand it. I am now defensive and always stick up for her as I know mine are very real and out of my control. The paramedics always think I'm drunk (despite my friends and blood tests telling them otherwise). And they slap the intoxicated label on—it's amazing how differently you're treated when people think it's self-inflicted.

I have had four episodes. All episodes were during a night out after alcohol, all were in a club, and all were associated with some form of high emotion. All gave me a Glasgow Coma Scale of 3/15, needing a nasopharyngeal airway and oxygen—on the fourth episode, a catheter (in resus ["resus," or the "trauma" area, is for seriously ill or injured patients with immediately life-threatening illnesses and injuries] for nine hours unresponsive) that then give me an *E. coli* urinary tract infection and a horrible post-ictal-like state. People judge you and dismiss it as fake. I am sick of people thinking I just can't handle my drink because I am sensible and responsible. I even went to my neurological consultant who thought that they were dissociative seizures that were caused by alcohol, as alcohol puts your mind in a subconscious state and doesn't want to deal with the overwhelming stress and so shuts off. My friends all have said that I've been sober and fine, then start being weird, then fall or just drop to the floor! The first two episodes, I had no warning, but the third and fourth times, I remember telling my friends that I felt weird, then I woke up in resus. I can recall odd parts of being in the ambulance or in the Accident and Emergency Department etc. but felt either confused or paralyzed. My mum said that they were applying so much pressure that my sternum was bruised purple, but I did not respond—if it was fake, then there is no way that I could put up with that pain and not flinch. My friend said she felt my heart rate and that it was absolutely racing. I remember all of a sudden feeling panicked, sweaty, and dizzy, and saying I couldn't move (after my friend had told me about her recent miscarriage and we were making friends after a recent falling out), then I woke up in resus again (this was on my twenty-seventh birthday).

I still am trying to find another diagnosis as I have many other confirmed health problems, including asthma, irritable bowel syndrome, endometriosis, heart valve regurgitation, chronic fatigue syndrome, neck and back pain, etc. They are wondering if it may be a result of something underlying, such as Lyme disease. But it takes months to get seen. So until then, I will have to either not drink or go clubbing, or wait until my next episode.

16

Person with PNES, UK

How has functional neurological disorders affected my life and me? Honestly, it has turned it upside down. Since being diagnosed, or even before that, I have felt frustrated. Constantly frustrated. I don't know what is going to trigger anything, what will happen next, when, on what day. I can't plan anything, and I certainly can't do the things that I used to enjoy doing. It plays havoc on my social life, my relationships with family and friends, my education and workload, and basically has put a massive barrier up for the rest of my life. To be honest, it's nice that I get to write all this as no one really asks or takes it into consideration, which is understandable, as I don't expect them to understand. I don't want sympathy as I am the sort of person that will push myself to my limits to help anyone out; however, in the last year, I have had to take a step back as I physically, emotionally, and mentally cannot do so. Again, FRUSTRATION!

With regard to professionals, I feel that out of all the "-ists" as I put it (neurologist, cardiologist, psychologist), no one seems to want to listen, or show a great deal of care. Put it this way, I was diagnosed and within two minutes was out of the clinic room after having been discharged as there was nothing they could do. Talk about being left in the dark. I actually searched my illness on the internet and found out about it through a functional neurological disorder website. I also joined a support group on Facebook where thousands of people have also had the same trouble from across the world. Not good really, *discriminative* is a word that comes to mind against health professionals who push you aside as you only have "functional problems." Yesterday, to be fair, I came across a psychologist who was amazing. Although she did not have much knowledge of functional neurological disorders apart from what she had to search on the internet, she sat back and listened and understood that I did not need support from the mental health team but physiology therapy [physical therapy] and occupational therapy. In her words, there is no point putting a plaster over a wound as it won't heal it. So my hopes are raised a little more with the extra help that I may receive (but I won't hold my breath).

Then we get on to relationships. Well, my husband has not got a clue as he has offered no support to me either. I swear, he thinks that I just have a cold sometimes, or the flu. Does not quite understand what is going on or how he is supposed to help. It has put so much added pressure on us, to the brink of a divorce nearly. Family are lovely, but the complete opposite. They don't like me doing anything, which is more frustrating as I'm not the type of person who can just sit there. Friends find it hard to accept that I can't always go out when things are planned as I don't know how I'll feel one day to the next. I had to defer from university as I couldn't concentrate, get assignments in on time, or sit in the same position through lectures. Although I plan to return in September, I believe a lot of support and adaptations are going to be needed; however, they are more than happy to help. I'm just super scared and anxious about returning and the thought of failing.

Symptoms come and go; the scariest is paralysis. I also have a heart condition, so when these symptoms do occur, I panic, which then sets off my heart. I lose balance, I'm only allowed plastic cutlery (as my husband moans that I'm breaking too much glass), and stairs and me don't go together. I can't sit for long, nor stand, nor walk. I can't sleep properly. Loud noises and lights affect me, and I'm constantly cold to the point I sometimes turn blue. My speech goes, and I stumble and slur. But again, it's frustrating as no health professional has given me any ideas or support to manage these symptoms. I feel very let down and even more so lonely.

It is a very lonely illness; half the time you don't know if it's your mind playing tricks or just because your brain does not want to know today. Proper messed up!!!! And then the big question! What does my life entail now? Well, I love my career with a passion, but I know that I can't watch children develop day in and day out as I can't work a five-day week. My only goal in life has been taken, and I cannot do anything I enjoy. I really do hate it.

17

Person with PNES, UK

My thoughts about having multiple seizures a day are not positive ones. Not only do they make me feel tired and groggy, but it also affects my mood. I feel angry all the time because I don't know or understand why it is happening to me. I find it hard to feel happy going to places I love and doing things that I love to do.

The seizures have affected my relationship with many people, including my ex-boyfriend. We were together for two years, but the stress of dealing with my seizures, the hospital trips, and all the ambulances called were too much for him to cope with, so he finished me.

I have had mental issues from a young age, which is one of the reasons why I can't figure out why the seizures started when they did. If the cause for them is psychological, then why didn't they start sooner? Why not in school when I went through so much pain, both physically and mentally, because of the bullying? My time in school was hell, and I am glad that I never have to go back.

I have had many thoughts about harming myself because of the seizures and how they make me feel. I do self-harm, but I have no attempted suicides. They stick at just being thoughts. I have seen the effects of someone committing suicide and what it does to the family. My aunty did exactly that, and I have blamed myself every day since.

Since I started with the seizures, my confidence has got less and less. I am afraid to leave the house most days because I don't know if anything is going to happen. I used to be active and do sports and go to the gym, but I am no longer allowed to go to my gym because of health and safety. When I attended the local college, I had to have a one-on-one support worker with me everywhere I went from entering the building to leaving. This made me feel like a child and not an eighteen-year-old. I have had so many different types of therapy over the last seven years, and I don't feel as though any of them truly helped me. I have also been on many different medications for depression, anxiety, migraines, and pain. Just like the therapies,

I don't feel as though the anti-anxiety medication did anything for me, but still I have to take it.

What my aunty did really affected me and still does today. I can't help but blame myself for her death. Did I make her stressed? Did I worry or scare her too much/ often? Should I have opened up to her the way that I did?

I can't help but think that maybe if I hadn't then she wouldn't have killed herself, and instead she wouldn't have had to worry about my problems.

18

Person with PNES, UK

I have a twin sister, so why hasn't she got this condition? I like to call it a condition rather than disorder or illness. It seems kinder. I remember attending a very quick discussion with a therapist, and she referred to the seizures as episodes and attacks. I dislike both these descriptions. Call it what it is—a seizure!! Don't sugarcoat the word. Truth be known, I don't fully understand why I seize. I look the same as my twin sister—why is it that I feel the weak one?? I hate what I have. It has destroyed what I had.

I have lost my driving license (my independence). There was no mention of non-epileptic attack disorder, and I had to contact the Driver and Vehicle Licensing Agency about it. Needless to say, they had not heard of it—epilepsy/seizure; same thing I was told. This is what I have found to be the case—people who witness my seizures say the same thing—looks like an epileptic fit. I find that I have to explain what non-epileptic attack disorder is. Again, that awful word *attack* is on here. I prefer NES (non-epileptic seizures). A disorder of the brain sounds quite worrying. It makes me feel like faulty goods. Each time I was asked to attend an occupational health assessment at my workplace, I seized. (I am currently on sick leave and unable to return to my job as a legal secretary.) I have asked to have a telephone discussion on each occasion but was denied my wish.

I remember coming around from one just after fifty minutes, not knowing where I was. I was on the floor with a pillow under my head! I also recalled hearing someone say "It's such a shame they have that" as I slowly came out of my seizure. That hurt. I've suddenly become "they." Who are "they"? I seized talking to my manager while on the phone. So concerned was the person that they contacted me again at 6 p.m. I've had a seizure lasting an hour and fifty minutes. Unfortunately, my seizures lengthened from forty minutes to an hour and forty-five minutes to two hours. My longest one has been two hours and twenty minutes. I have no idea of the passing of time. Consequently, Human Resources would not allow me back into work. My union has become involved. My workplace has no understanding of the condition. I was offered a buddy and part-time work as a resettle adjustment. But as my consultant says, it doesn't work like that, which is exactly what I told my boss. I have only learned that I've been given "ill health–retirement." I'm happy with the decision, but I'm extremely sad that I've lost my job. It was a good company, with good colleagues and friends. I shall miss the banter and the laughs we had. I've worked there since leaving school. I should have retired properly from there. I'm still relatively young.

Sometimes I get a warning—shaking of my hands or a sudden rush in my head of little waves of pressure (I can only liken this to sitting up too quickly or spinning round and round and how suddenly stopping makes you feel dizzy). I have what I call my huge head waves, which usually knock me off my feet and I fall. These are the ones where I injure myself. I've had carpet burns, bruises galore, sprained neck, bitten tongue, cuts, and scars to prove it. I've seized in company, which leaves me embarrassed. I hate people seeing me like that, I care about these people, and I don't like to know that I've caused distress or made them alarmed. One family member won't stay in my company for longer than ten minutes. It's sad on my part. I feel different from other people. I seize watching the television, having a cup of tea, doing a crossword, all mundane things. My self-esteem is low. I have seen little of my friends, even though they have been nice. I don't want them to see me like that; it's not nice for them. I seized at the doctor's surgery ["doctor's surgery" is where general practitioners see patients] after a twenty-five-minute wait; I was told they called the ambulance. I was rudely taken out of my seizure by a paramedic slapping my face on both sides and intentionally shouting down my ear "Do you know where you are?" I could not focus on his face, I was so dazed, stop looking up here I'm down here, here, here. The hospital didn't read the bracelet I was wearing nor did the paramedic, but in my head, I feel I'd have been asked, "Non-epileptic attack disorder, what is that?"

19

Person with PNES, UK

Before I had my seizures, I was able to go out by myself with confidence; I was able to do anything I wanted. Yes—I struggled because I had my fibromyalgia and headaches, but I had my independence. Now I feel like I can't go out many places alone, if anywhere; if I do go out alone, it's to the corner shop with my phone or getting a taxi to somewhere that people know me because I cannot get the bus alone. It is not just me who thinks that I cannot do these things, it is the people around me; they do not trust that I can cope or that I am well enough now that I have these seizures to do things alone. I know that they are coming from a good place, I really do, but sometimes, just sometimes, I wish that they would grant me a little bit more freedom.

I've found that many people do not understand the nature of these kinds of seizures and of course that is bound to affect my relationships with them. I have distanced myself from these people feeling that if I don't understand it properly myself, then how on earth can I explain it to them. This leaves them wondering if they have done something wrong (which of course is nothing), and ultimately, our friendships and family ties have suffered greatly as a result.

Daily or nearly daily seizures have of course meant that I am unable to work; also, the fatigue that this causes is so relentless that I feel had I found an understanding employment situation, I simply would just be too tired. This leaves me living off state benefits, and I do not see an end in sight where I can come off them. I would love to do so many things in my life, but they all need money, and this is money that I cannot acquire. I want to travel, get married, make my flat look nice, etc. About traveling, I can't even do that because of my seizures. I struggle to travel on a bus or car for any distance without a seizure coming on, so this puts me and my partner off traveling very far, leaving us isolated.

I am now twenty-six and living with the man that I want to spend the rest of my life with. Before I met him, I didn't think that I'd be able to find any man who could handle all of my illnesses as it had been a breaking point in other relationships, but now I know that he can handle it. I just hope that my seizures and illnesses won't get in the way of our life and hopefully our plans to start a family.

A LETTER TO MY NON-EPILEPTIC SEIZURES

This feels strange writing to you as you are now a part of me. It's like I'm writing to myself. There are so many things that I have to say, so many things I feel like you have impacted on my life (the good and the bad), so excuse me if this comes out a rambling mess because these things are the things I have left unsaid.

When I was first diagnosed with fibromyalgia, that was a devastating blow. I was only twenty-one or twenty-two, and I had so much I wanted to do. I carried on, though. I changed my path a little, only accepting part-time jobs, but I carried on. Little did I know that a year later, these seizures would attack me with full force after taking time off sick for other illnesses. I wish you could have warned me that functional neurological disorder and non-epileptic attack disorder were connected. I wish there had been some awareness because I was left out in the dark, floundering, looking for answers that would have made things so much easier for me and my family.

The first time I had a big seizure, I can only remember what I was told, but by all accounts, you took a lot of my dignity away from me. I lost all awareness of who I was; I couldn't even remember my name or date of birth between seizures. I repeatedly lost consciousness and even began to lash out in anger, and what I can only imagine now was some kind of visual hallucination. All I can remember about the situation is being scared. How is it right that you do that to a young woman, how does she deserve this level of torture?

Over the years, my seizures have improved and then gotten worse again. One of the hardest things to see is that people don't understand because you are not a real illness. My pain I experience when part of my body seizes is ridiculous, and you do that to me—I'm always left wondering, why me?

On the other hand, I want to thank you because without you I probably wouldn't have met the man that I'm in love with now. You see, you knocked my confidence down so much that the thought of speaking to a man face-to-face was beyond me, so I turned to a dating website to talk to people and build myself up, not expecting to meet the man of my dreams, my future husband.

Through having seizures, I have also been pushed to be honest with myself and my family about things that have happened in the past. I was hopeful that this might help you go away, but no luck yet. But at least it is helpful in keeping me happy and stopping me from putting things to one side like usual.

When I was first diagnosed, the doctors were quick to say that the reason behind you was that I had recently been told I needed brain surgery, which was subsequently cancelled, but the idea of it has been broached again, so I am scared, scared that you are ready to pounce like the bad dog that you are and attack with your full force again.

If I want you to remember anything from this letter, it is that you take away from people and leave them with fear, and for to me, that is your biggest power. In the future, I want to be strong enough not to be scared of you because, like I said, you are a part of me, and you can't be scared of your own shadow.

20

Person with PNES, UK

I have quite a few seizures per day. The official diagnosis for my seizures is non-epileptic attack disorder. It is believed that they are connected to stress and panic, which I am dealing with in high levels at present and have done so for some time. In short, I am a single mother to a sixteen-year-old, my father suffers from dementia, and I was married to a man who unfortunately turned out to be an alcoholic who repeatedly abused me mentally, physically, and sexually during our whole fifteen-year relationship. This ended in divorce due to physical violence ten years ago. However, my ex-husband does not admit to doing anything wrong and continues to this day attempting to contact me on any occasion possible using anything, including the house and our daughter, as a way to gain some sort of reaction from me. Things of course go deeper than I have time to write, but I think that these events have led to what I believe are severe attacks caused by stress and panic.

The way these seizures make me feel is this: Until recently, genuinely, I believed that I was indeed dying. It has taken my doctor sending me for another brain scan at my request to convince me that I do not have a fatal brain disease. I try not to let the seizures prevent me from doing anything. I go out every day shopping, even though I often have a seizure when I am out. I have become very adept at disguising when I am having one. They only last a matter of moments, and I do not think that I could cope with anyone fussing around me to see if I was okay. I have seizures when I am confronted with the slightest thing, even a simple telephone call or conversation, so you could say that I have a fear of confrontation. I have had therapy, which I found helpful as I learned to explore my own self-worth, and I have come to realize that I am indeed a person in my own right, a very intelligent one. Also, I learned several useful breathing tips to help deal with stress, which I encounter on a daily basis.

The seizures that I have are frequent but do not last long. They make me feel like a lesser person. Indeed, I thought for years that I had epilepsy, and it comes as somewhat of a relief that these seizures can and are controlled by me personally, without the need for medication (most of them, that is). I find that they are worse when I attempt to relax, and so they are more severe at bedtime. I do not find relaxing easy; it is not something that I am used to doing. I did not find therapy easy at all because it meant looking into my feelings and past, something that I buried. I am not a person that is used to delegating anything to anyone. I have always been a person who has been controlled, especially by men, my entire life.

I try not to let my seizures affect my independence. I often go out alone as when I am near others it signals confrontation of some sort. When it comes to a fight-or-flight response, I am constantly in flight mode. I never relax. I find it very difficult to do so. However, if I allowed it, my friends and family would not let me go out anywhere without them. I feel trapped all the time. I constantly feel something bad is about to happen. I lost my mother three years ago to a sudden stroke that I believe was in part caused by stress. She went to bed one night and never woke up. We had to switch off her life support machine in the next couple of days. I think her death had more of an effect on everyone than what was admitted. My father, who now has dementia and is somewhat a control freak, is a difficult man to say the least. His care has largely fallen to me. I believe that my symptoms are physiological and will lessen when my stress levels are allowed to reduce.

21

Person with Epilepsy and PNES, UK

Living with seizures alone is hard work, but believe it or not, living with epileptic seizures and non-epileptic seizures is even harder. Sometimes they are hard to tell apart, but other times they are completely different. Some people themselves wouldn't be able to understand, even family, and neither did I at one point in my life. Before all of this, I was completely oblivious.

Dealing with seizures affects my life terribly. I don't have the independence I'd like or the confidence. I also have to be with someone, not only for the fact of maybe having a seizure, but just to feel safe.

I also deal with absences, which from what I've learned from previous consultants are partial seizures. They cause me to completely blank out, yet I can move around. I move things, pick things up, and put them in my mouth. I can become a danger to people around me, and I have absolutely no control. The aftermath of these types of seizures make me very fatigued, I just sleep for numerous hours, feeling sick, and I have no appetite. This can carry on for days on end after each partial seizure.

The difference between non-epileptic and epileptic seizures is that I sometimes notice I can be tired. Some I seem to recover from a lot faster than I do from others, which makes me wonder if it could have possibly been non-epileptic or epileptic. With non-epileptic seizures, I don't lose control (e.g., I don't wet myself during one, nor do I dribble or foam at the mouth). I don't always take as long to come around after the seizure either, but with epileptic seizures, all these things occur. Before I was diagnosed with non-epileptic seizures, I didn't notice these differences. I just assumed it was an unusual epileptic seizure, and I carried on thinking so until I told my consultant these changes, to which he finally found out the reason that I was experiencing both types of seizures.

I have non-epileptic seizures mostly due to having bad anxiety, and instead of the panic or anxiety attacks, I go into a seizure instead. I don't have any signs before either seizure; I just fall where I am.

There are many differences between the seizures, yet unfortunately, they both have the same outcome. They can be hard to control, like mine are at the moment, and are difficult to live with and can be dangerous. It's hard for my family to have to live with them as well, seeing me in such a vulnerable state most of the time, unable to help, which is also out of their own control.

It's even hard trying to explain these things to people who don't understand seizures at all, never mind the differences.

22

Person with PNES, UK

I have an appointment with an audiologist because I think that I have hyperacusis. I find it almost unbearable being in large crowds because of the noise, and I also find it hard to cope with loud noises and high-pitched sounds. It has in the past caused quite a few non-epileptic attacks, and I have ended up in the hospital because of it.

As I am off work at the moment, I have to find things to do to pass the time. I have had a busy week because my friend has been off with me. Last Monday, I walked into the city center to get some exercise as I hadn't done any in a few days and exercise makes me feel better. The walk is about three miles in total. I went to get a videogame for my computer as I find playing video games relaxes me and keeps my mind focused so I don't feel lonely or upset about my current situation. I was sacked about four weeks ago from another job (I think this is job number four now) because of my non-epileptic attack disorder. Over the last few weeks, I have been reflecting on my triggers and trying to assess how best to cope with this condition. It was only about a month ago that I accepted the fact that I have this condition. I know that my triggers are related to noise and crowds, and feeling trapped, so this is why I find that solitude calms me down.

For the past couple of months, I have been seeing a therapist. I have a lot of unresolved emotions that cause my non-epileptic seizures, so she helps me with this. I have had a lot of trauma in my life and was on antidepressants for a long time, which did not help my situation at all.

On Wednesday, my best friend and I went to my parents' caravan [in the UK, a caravan is a mobile home typically used for vacations] in the countryside for a couple of days. I am at my most peaceful when I am in nature. For the couple of days that we were there, we went on a few walks and relaxed. When I am in a place of peace and among nature, it resets my body so I can cope with daily life again.

On Friday, when I arrived home, I went to see a comedian with my parents and my boyfriend as a present to my dad. It was a really good night, and we had lots of laughs. I find laughter calms me down as well.

On Saturday, I went to the caravan with my parents and my boyfriend again, and we had a lovely weekend. My mum doesn't know that I went with my friend during the week because she still thinks that I am working. I find it is best not to tell her about my current situation because I don't want to worry her. I don't like lying to her, but it is the better of the two situations and causes me the least amount of stress.

23

Person with PNES, USA

In June 2015, I was officially diagnosed with psychogenic non-epileptic seizures, after having them since November 2010. Before this time, I was told that I had conversion disorder, but I was given no help to address the underlying causes of the disorder other than high doses of epileptic seizure medicine.

Before an episode, I dissociate. It is an out-of-body experience. I know that I'm in my body, but I'm not connected to it. I feel foggy in my brain—there is a light-headed "about to pass out" feeling that washes over me, and a drop sensation. I become EXTREMELY tired. Sometimes I have enough of these warnings to sit down; other times I am caught completely off guard and will fall to the floor. Falling used to bother me—now I almost want to fall over or sit because it gives me some kind of grounding. During the episode, when they are at their worst, my hands and feet will go cold. I have told my family about this, and they are able to rub my hands and put blankets on my feet. Also, in the more severe ones, I will range from mild ticks/jerks to severe convulsing and repetitive face movement. It is exhausting. I have never lost consciousness or continence during an episode; I am always able to hear what is going on, and though my eyes cross, I can see and keep track of who is around me. If I am startled, my startle reflex is high. I've learned to do deep breathing when I can concentrate on that and to let the episode run its course. My episodes range from five minutes to two hours. I've learned that it depends on the trigger and vulnerability factors preceding the episode (was I hungry, tired, did I miss a medication, etc.). After the episode, I am ALWAYS exhausted. I usually come out of it and go straight to bed. Sometimes it takes me thirty minutes to regain the strength to even walk—other times I am able to shuffle to bed right away. I will fall asleep for hours. To me, it feels like my body has just been through a marathon, and I have to rest to catch up with what has taken place.

The unpredictable nature of the episodes can be very frustrating. I have learned a lot of self-patience with these episodes and try to speak kindly to myself when I am suffering. My family has been the biggest source of support during my episodes. They hold my neck up, cover me in blankets, rub my hands, and are just there. It is so comforting to have them nearby when I can't do anything for myself. I have had to explain many times to friends about what to expect, that I am okay and I can hear them, and to please just give me the time/space to let the episode finish. OH! And to NOT call 911 [the emergency number for the US], for an ambulance! There is nothing the hospital can do for me because I know the episodes are not epileptic, so I just have to let it run its course. I've only had a few episodes around my friends, and they have all been good about letting me be. Sometimes the fear of someone calling 911 makes the episode worse.

My first-ever episode in 2010 was horrible. It was confusing and traumatic. I know that everyone there was trying to do their best, but it was really hard to have the emergency medical technicians say what they were seeing was "weird." And in 2014, while having another EEG, I heard a technician say that I was "faking it." That hurt. A lot. Because in my mind, I thought, "Why would I fake this? Why would I want to be unable to move for minutes to hours? How is this fun or reinforcing for me?" Neurologists and psychiatrists have thrown me back and forth to each other—each not knowing what to do and figuring that the other party would know. It was so painful to not have a place to go for help. No one knew what to do with me. And I felt so out of place.

A few times during the past six years I wanted to end my life because having these episodes was not how I wanted to live. Luckily, I was treated for that and do not feel that way now. I have found that the episodes come and go in waves. From 2010 to the present, I had a brief, fourteen-month period of independence where I was working and living on my own. When the episodes kicked up, I had to move back home with my family for help. My independence has taken a huge hit, and financially, I have had to rely on my parents. This has been especially scary when it came to insurance coverage after I turned twenty-six. I am a Speech Therapist Assistant but had to quit my job when my depression/episodes became worse. I was able to take a fourteen-hour-a-week job in the evenings over the last year and have successfully worked there for almost a year! This is a huge accomplishment. My goal is to return to Speech Therapy this year. I never thought this would happen. It is a huge blessing for me.

For a long time, I hated myself. I felt doomed to this punishment that I didn't understand—and that professionals didn't understand either. I felt completely out of control. I turned to self-harming to try and cope with the painful feelings. After my first hospitalization, I found dialectical behavioral therapy. **It has changed my life.** My thinking is different, my coping skills are better, I can problem solve situations, and most importantly, my counselor and I have worked together to address the traumatic events that happened right before my episodes began. Three different psychiatrists could not figure out what the "big traumatic event" was—I wasn't raped, I didn't go to war, etc. It wasn't big and obvious, and so they weren't sure what was wrong with me. When I began telling my counselor about specific events that happened before my first episode in 2010, we both realized that those were traumatic for me. And that has been one of the greatest things that I have learned: What is traumatic for one person may not/will not be traumatic for another. My events were a series of "smaller" (if we want to use that word) events that continuously picked at me. I was already vulnerable and sensitive—predisposed—to feeling/acting/responding in certain ways, and these events pushed my mind over the edge to where shutting down was the only way my mind/body could figure out how to get me out of the current situation and get some serious help. It's okay—and normal—if your traumatic events are different than others. We are all different, so what affects one person one way may not affect another person in the same way.

When my episodes started six years ago, I felt out of control, at a loss, and a complete failure. Now, SO many things have changed. I am doing prolonged exposure therapy to directly address the trauma. I continue to attend weekly dialectical behavior therapy sessions to learn coping skills and map out my triggers so I can change the events after I am triggered instead of shutting down. I have added in trauma yoga, where I am able to release the extra energy that builds up in my system so I don't go into shutdown mode (episode mode) but am able to handle reality on reality's terms. And I saw the biggest change when I started seeing an eastern medicine doctor of chiropractic who uses a special technique (called neuromodulation technique) to HEAL my body. It has been a miracle to watch. My thinking has changed, my health has changed, my coping skills have changed, and because of all of this, I am able to react differently to the episodes when they come. I thought psychogenic non-epileptic seizures was a doomed diagnosis, but I have found that with a lot of hard work and a team of "out of the box" professionals who BELIEVE in me, I am going to be able to live a normal, productive, life worth living.

24

Person with Epilepsy and PNES, USA

I don't like them. I hate my seizures with a passion because nobody believes me. Every time I have one, I feel that people judge me. It's very frustrating to me that when I had an EEG test done, they said that there was indication of seizure activity, but then the discharge papers said there were no seizures. Having non-epileptic seizures is hard for me because of the lack of understanding and the fact that the process of trying to educate people is difficult as it feels to me like people don't want to be educated. When I feel a seizure coming, I am sometimes afraid to tell people because I am afraid that they won't take it seriously. That is a scary feeling. My friends and family understand what it is like for me and try to support me as best they can. One friend even says, "I know it is something you don't have control over."

25

Person with PNES, UK

I was diagnosed with dissociative seizures well over ten years ago. When I first started to have them, I was extremely scared and alone. The typical response was "She is doing this for attention," or "It's all in her head." I can tell you now that this made me isolate myself; I hid in shame and was embarrassed to leave the house. The doctors say it's not epilepsy; we need to refer you to hospital, so I doubted myself, I wondered if I was going mad. No one seemed to understand or be able to explain it.

I recall once when I was pregnant and my partner's mum called an ambulance as I had been seizing for five hours straight, they feared for the safety of my unborn child. I was in and out of consciousness, and I can recall the paramedic asking my partner at the time, "Is she epileptic?" He replied no, so they then asked if I had taken dugs. I was mortified. On arrival at the hospital, they stuck me on the labor ward and just left me. I pleaded for a fan as I felt my head was burning, I was told that I was being silly and that I was actually quite cold. It took my partner to get angry for them to finally, an hour later, provide me with a fan. I left feeling gutted and uncared for, but mostly I felt branded a fake and a liar.

Over the next few months, I met a professor who explained to me that I was not alone and in fact this was quite common. This professor explained to me that emotions are a type of energy, and as I stored them in my head, they built up, like little sparks of electricity; over time, the ball of electricity gets bigger and bigger, and then one day, it has to be released . . . cue seizures. This made things a bit clearer; however, with little support other than him, which was once very few months, I was still at this time very alone. I was referred to psychotherapeutic counseling with a waiting list of at least six months.

Getting help doesn't happen fast. Back in my day, and still today, really it was all so new to the general practitioner, no information, no advice or help readily available. Doctors referred to it as a type of depression, and I remember one doctor saying, "It's all in your head, just keep telling yourself that you're okay and you will be," which over ten years later and telling myself this . . . I am okay, I am just still having seizures.

I recall a friend asking me once what should she do if I was to have a seizure. I felt quite heartfelt that someone should care enough to ask, only to have some smart aleck shout, "Run a hot bath and put her in it, then add the washing!" When you're already isolated and feeling low about yourself, this is the last thing you need, people mocking you, but in time, you learn to ignore their ignorance.

So how do I feel when I have a seizure? Usually, I become distant in my head, foggy and unresponsive. I hear you, but you're echoing and seem blurred. My head burns like it's on fire. My body shakes violently and uncontrollably, I become dry mouthed, tired, and my eyes sometimes roll back. I can hear people; however, I can't make the words come out of my mouth, my arms and legs become achy, and my hands sometimes clench. I often lose the use of my legs and sometimes my hands. The pain is like being electrocuted from the brain down through my spine. I do not always remember what has happened, and in fact, my memory to this day is beyond terrible—I have to write everything down. Luckily for me, I can sign British Sign Language, so I communicate to my family this way when I can. I find the worst thing anyone can do around me when I have a seizure is to talk about it or me; this heightens my sensors to the issues and creates panic in my head, making things worse. I find just aiding me with sips of cold water, a cool fan, and ensuring that I am safe is the best help anyone can give. Talking about other things to take my mind off it and helping me to relax is also useful.

The hardest thing about a seizure is that I find I need to empty my body, so I need frequent trips to the toilet, which isn't always easy when your body is violently shaking and you have lost the use of your legs. Before he passed away, my husband would carry me to the toilet. After a seizure, it can take days to regain my strength, I have a massive loss of appetite, and my memory is at its worst. I have little long-term memory left. My body aches like I have been in a fight, I usually have bruising all over, and I feel very weak. Simple tasks become harder to do, and I even break down and cry over silly things. I recall having a complete meltdown one Sunday as someone had stolen my Yorkshire puddings from the oven; my daughter then pointed out that I was looking in the washing machine. I just sat and cried; I felt like I was going mad.

When I was awaiting the diagnosis, and even after I was diagnosed, the rude comments and negative medical responses made me become very isolated. This caused severe anxiety, which over the years has worsened.

I avoid any social interaction, events, and gatherings unless I have someone that I feel safe with. I was so bad at one point in my life that I refused to leave the house full stop. But good friends took me on small trips out to the supermarket and to local places to help me overcome this. Still, to this day, I will not go anywhere alone unless it is local and I feel safe. I cannot do the food shopping unless I have an adult with me; I cannot travel to new places or plan trips out unless, again, I have someone with me and I have planned it to the dot. I have become very obsessive-compulsive; I cannot cope with surprises or anything unplanned or unexpected. I am now a widow and have four children; sadly, this affects their lives as I won't travel far, so they miss out on so much. This riddles me with guilt. I have no family other than them, so I feel very alone.

If I'm honest, my illness has affected past relationships. I have always felt like a burden and as if I didn't deserve to be loved. I have become very hard-hearted and prefer my own company. I have purposely pushed people away to save them the trouble of having to be with me, at my own cost of heartbreak. My husband was the first person to see past my seizures and was just as stubborn as I am. He wasn't fond of trips out like me, so we enjoyed time at home making our garden special. Now, though, I don't have him, so it's a very lonely world. I have become a prisoner of my own mind. Trapped in a world of shame and self-doubt.

With the social media network expanding, there are now many support groups for people suffering seizures. Not everyone on them is helpful, but most are and usually help and offer advice to support you. Over time, you will learn through no choice but to deal and cope with your seizures, and you will through experience understand what suits your needs the best. Everyone is an individual, however, but now thanks to some great people, we are no longer alone.

How do I cope? I ask myself this question all the time, and if I'm honest, I don't, but through experience and time, I have learned to take it as it comes. It's going to happen no matter how hard I try and stop it. So rather than worry about it now, I try to enjoy a quiet life. I do not drink alcohol, and have not for many years, as I found that this worsens the seizures. I avoid anything that makes me uncomfortable, busy places for example, and I go to bed early to ensure plenty of rest. I plan my shopping trips around having someone with me, and I plan events such as Christmas months in advance to avoid busy shops and chaos.

I do not work as I care for my disabled daughter and I also have other illnesses myself; however, when I did, I found that I was unable to work in busy places. I could not use a computer for long periods of time as this would trigger a seizure, too much stress would be a trigger, tiredness too. In my spare time, I found that I cannot go into places like clubs due to the lights and noise of too many people, busy enclosed shopping centers, buses, and attractions, like fairs and amusement parks, due to the rides setting me off. I have found that I have not been able to cope in the cinema due to the lighting of certain films. I have also noticed a change in my vision since my seizures started. It has worsened, dramatically. I was advised to stop having baths as they trigger a seizure, so now I only shower. Every person is different obviously, but these are the things that I would avoid. Having dissociative seizures has ruined my life; I dream of just going somewhere, anywhere, no plans, no worries, but it isn't going to happen. So I try and find the positives in it, and I try and make my life as happy as I can.

The hardest part of it all is the loneliness, and I guess some of that is my own fault, by pushing people away to save myself embarrassment, avoiding situations like weddings, etc. I have recently restarted my psychotherapeutic counseling with the hope to again find a way to help me understand and somehow control my seizures. The more the medical world learns and understands about this illness, the more I jump in and try to learn too. Recently, I took part in a study to see if writing about them helped. When I wrote about my day as it was to be, I found I felt worse, and I panicked more about what was going to be; however, I found when I wrote about the day after it took place, I could find positives in how I handled my day and seizures. I am currently trying to alter my flight-or-fight response in my brain. I have discovered that if I face a situation that I really want to run from, then slowly, over time, it becomes less of a problem. This is very hard to do, but it's something that I am focusing on at the moment.

Which brings me to my final discovery—I cannot sit still. I have found that having dissociative seizures, I am unable to relax. I have found I need to be constantly busy, and I will not stop until I collapse. I have tried mindfulness, and again, I felt agitated. It is as if I need my mind to be active at all times. When it comes to sleeping, I struggle; it's like my brain will not switch off. I have vivid dreams and wake in cold sweats, scared and shaking.

My advice to anyone who has dissociative seizures: do not let it make you depressed, turn the tables around, study it, read about it, find others who suffer from it, and make it your sole target to fully understand it. We are not fakers, attention seekers, or anything else people throw at us. We are human beings with feelings and needs. And the more we learn about it, the more others will understand.

26

Person with PNES, UK

I hate my seizures and my chronic fatigue syndrome. My mental illness is something that I can cope with, but being worried all the time if I'm going to have a seizure if I go anywhere (which I usually do) is unbearable—it has made me not want to leave the house.

My seizures were so bad in the beginning that I missed both my children's most important teen years when they were growing up and they needed me. But I was unable to be there for them; having a neurological illness on top of the seizures gives me extra pain and spasms. It all makes my quality of life pretty low—I need help with things like bathing, dressing, washing my hair, cooking, and looking after my money.

My husband used to take care of me, but it was too much for him and he left, which killed me.

I have been a bulimic since I was twelve, and my medication has made me put on over four stone [fifty-six pounds], which has made me so depressed, and I hate myself even more. I am a self-harmer, mainly cutting my belly, which I hate because it is fat from medication! I get so embarrassed if I have a seizure in public or even around people I know. They have stopped me from driving, and I can't have my grandchildren on my own in case I have a seizure. I don't go out because I don't want people who knew me before I was ill to see me or in case I have a seizure in front of them—I can see the look on their faces of disgust.

27

Person with PNES, UK

In June 2015, I was admitted to the hospital following a severe asthma attack. After several treatment attempts, I was given an infusion. Two days after the infusion, I started to have seizures. They started off as a faint, with minor trembling, but quickly escalated into full tonic-clonic seizures, and I was having over twenty a day. Following a consultation, it was decided that I was having a rare side effect from the medication associated with the infusion, and the infusion was stopped. After a week of no infusions, I was still suffering the seizures - they were still severe and frequent. I spent seven weeks in the hospital with a combination of asthma and seizures, during which time numerous tests were done, including an electroencephalogram, electrocardiogram, and various scans. All the tests were coming back negative, and I was growing extremely concerned and frightened, and so I started doing my own research. I entered seizures into a search engine and started to read.

One of the results referred to non-epileptic attack disorder. I read up on this disorder, and it struck a chord with me. I had been suffering from severe asthma since 2005 (I'd had asthma prior to that, but it was easily controlled), which had been getting steadily worse, particularly during the summer. when my asthma is very brittle due to a severe grass pollen allergy. I was well aware that I had been struggling with my mood over the last few years, requiring medication in the form of anti-depressants. I also had a history of depression and anxiety from childhood, compounded by poor relationship choices, family relationship difficulties, and a serious assault resulting in post-traumatic stress disorder.

The diagnosis was confirmed by a neurological consultation during which I had a seizure. Prior to June, I was functioning, albeit sometimes not too well, as a contributing member of society. I had a full-time job; I was able to cope with difficult family relationships; I was able to maintain friendships and be there for people who needed me. Since the seizures started, this has all changed.

I no longer have any contact with most of my family, who are not able to understand what is going on and have made a difficult time even more difficult. I am currently not working. I only leave my flat to attend medical appointments, and I struggle to maintain friendships.

I spoke to my asthma team about the difficulties that I was experiencing and the impact this was having on my asthma. They wrote to my general practitioner and recommended counseling. My doctor sent off the referral, and I was warned that it would take some months before anyone would be available.

My experiences with the Accident and Emergency Department have been horrible. On one occasion, I was taken in by ambulance following a seizure. I had been in a few times previously, so some staff was aware of me. On arriving at the hospital, I was taken off the stretcher and put in to the main waiting room. I was there for approximately an hour when I had a further seizure. I came to surrounded by hospital staff; I then heard a nurse say, "Pseudo," and everyone left with the exception of one male nurse, who continued to assist me. Another nurse chastised him for remaining with me, and they both left. I was confused, upset, and frightened. I had just had a seizure, and I desperately needed to sleep. I knew that if I didn't, there was a high probability that I would have a further seizure fairly quickly, and I was sitting in the middle of a number of people who now thought that I was "faking" the whole thing. I was seen and admitted with a concussion.

On another occasion, very shortly after the seizures started, I woke up feeling extremely dizzy; I was unable to walk and felt really sick. I had never experienced these symptoms before, and I was concerned that I had hit my head during a seizure overnight. I rang 111 [the UK National Health Service non-emergency number] for some advice and they sent a paramedic out to see me. The paramedic was unsympathetic and made me feel like I was wasting his time; it was only after I staggered to the kitchen to vomit that he began to take a begrudging interest. Following the taking of my stats [vital signs] he called an ambulance. While waiting for the ambulance, I had a seizure. I came to on the floor (I had come off the sofa). Due to the position of my head, I was finding it very hard to breathe; the medic was standing there looking at me and told me to sit up and that I could control it. When the ambulance crew arrived, he did his handover and did everything but say that I was a time waster. If I hadn't felt so ill, I would have sent them all away, but I did not know what was going on. I was taken to the hospital and again placed in the waiting room. I was called through to triage, during which I had a seizure. Following the seizure, I was violently sick. I was admitted and was in for three days before the dizziness stopped. I am now aware that the dizziness and sickness is all part of the disorder. I do not call for help on these days, but I stay in bed until it passes, which can sometimes take a few days.

I try to avoid attending the Accident and Emergency Room for my seizures as often as I can, but I am normally quite out of it for a while and the decision is made for me. During my last attendance, I had a seizure in the exam room and came off the trolley; I came to on the floor with someone pinching my shoulder. This is not an unusual experience. I normally wake up to pain as this is the way that most medical professionals try to rouse you. I was being told to get up, but at that stage, I was still pretty out of it; the next thing I heard was "Well, I'm not picking you up, you can stay there." The female then left. Once I had roused myself, I moved so that I was sitting with my back to the wall. I was very distressed due to the aftereffects of the seizure and the treatment I had received. A nurse passing my room saw me and asked the desk (out of my sight) why I was on the floor; a female responded, "She put herself there, she is always throwing herself off things." I was distraught. I was actually trying to work out how I could get to the roof to throw myself off; I just couldn't take it any longer. My life was saved that day by the kindness of a porter. He saw me crying on the floor and came in to ask why I was sitting on the floor, and I told him I was too scared to get back on the trolley. He moved the trolley against the wall and put two chairs next to it so that if I did fall, I would land on them instead of the floor, it was such a simple thing, but it made a huge difference to me. He then went and made me a cup of tea.

During all this, I was reading everything I could. I bought a book on "Psychogenic Attack Disorder" and attempted a number of ways of self-help, including relaxation and mindfulness, with very little improvement. I needed help.

I had to wait six months to receive counseling, and after two sessions, it was decided that my symptoms were too severe and that I needed to be referred to see a psychologist, which would probably take another six months. My mood deteriorated, resulting in an overdose, following which I was admitted to a mental health hospital. I spent three months in there; I attended psychology and every class that was available in an attempt to get better. The classes were helpful, the psychology enlightening. It transpires that I have been using dissociation to deal with difficult situations since I was a child; the seizures would appear to be a worsening of this. After three months, it was decided that my issues were "long term" and would require further treatment in the community. I was no longer in crisis and was discharged.

I have been discharged with a community psychiatric nurse, who has been working with me to get a treatment plan in place. Obviously, the priority is to see a psychologist; unfortunately, there is a long delay on this. I have therefore been referred for art therapy in the meantime. Unfortunately, I am now in my peak allergy season, and my asthma has once again taken off. This has meant that I have been unable to attend the art classes. The seizures, which had gotten down to one to three a day, have increased; it is an egg-and-chicken question over which is triggering which.

I am an intelligent, sensible, and logical person. I can see what I am doing to myself. I understand the physical side of it, but no matter how hard I try, I cannot stop it.

This disorder has had a massive negative impact on my life. Add to that the lack of understanding within the medical profession (most notably Accident and Emergency nurses), the lack of availability of timely treatment, and you can understand why I still ask the question every day—is it worth it?

28

Person with PNES, UK

Living with non-epileptic seizures could be classed as pure hell OR you can turn that right around and say they changed my life. When I first had seizures, I was diagnosed with epilepsy, a diagnosis I never believed. I have no idea why, I used to tell people, I have seizures and that the doctors said it was epilepsy, but I knew it wasn't.

At the time my seizures started, I was living in a hellish situation where every day was a battle for survival. Six years later, I escaped that situation, and that very day, my seizures stopped. I got my driving license back, and I tried to get on with my life. I truly believed that I could get my life back on track. In reality, this was not the case, and my life was a constant battle. But at that stage, I thought I was normal and it was everyone else who had the problem.

When I woke up one morning and my dog was dead, my life fell apart, and it was that day that I knew I needed help before I went mad. I was invited to a cognitive behavioral therapy group at the mental health unit, but while everyone started moving forward, my life just continued to unravel. The psychologist who ran the group asked me some tough questions, and eventually, I opened up to her. I was at this point taken out of the group, offered trauma therapy, and diagnosed with post-traumatic stress disorder. The day I got that diagnosis, I felt like a weight had been lifted off of me . . . I wasn't going mad . . . I was ill. Three weeks into trauma therapy and I was found having a seizure; they had returned. A few weeks later, after a therapy session, I had multiple seizures and was taken to the doctors from therapy. The doctor had me admitted to the neurology ward. After four days on the ward and numerous tests, a man in a suit asked if he could sit next to my bed and talk. I said yes; I just wanted to go home. He introduced himself as a professor and told me that he had something to tell me that I may find difficult. He then went on to tell me that I didn't have epilepsy, but I did have non-epileptic seizures due to trauma. My response was "Excellent, so I can get better." After more talking, handouts, and a website address, I was allowed to go home. Once I had absorbed the information and what it meant, I cried, simply because other people had inflicted me with this condition and, after everything I had gone through, I still had a battle to live. I did, however, keep in mind that I CAN get better from this.

What can I say, life is difficult. I wake up on the floor, having relived my trauma, and I have no idea who anyone is or where I am. It is frightening, and the fear is unbelievable. I made my mind up that this was not going to stop me going out and living my life, and it hasn't. OK, some days I don't make it to my destination and end up at the hospital, but I go home, have a cry, and then get back on my feet and try again. This is a condition that can make you want to die, so you have to play it at its own game and not let it defeat you. Fifty percent of people can recover, they say, and I WILL be in that fifty percent!!! I have now completed two years of trauma therapy, and while at first I hated going, the therapist has helped me to turn my life around. She also diagnosed me with complex post-traumatic stress disorder. At the same time, I attended an adult college where they accepted the seizures and my complex post-traumatic stress disorder. One particular tutor at college, more than anything, changed my life and also saved my life. She helped me to learn to trust people again and showed me people do care. She also taught me that with hard work, I can overcome the past. It is not going to be easy, but I am getting there. I am currently at university, still having seizures, but living my life, and I hope in the future to conquer the seizures and work again.

Getting my life back is the ultimate revenge to those who destroyed it, but it is also a battle that has taught me so much about myself. I look back and say that if my trauma and the non-epileptic seizures hadn't ever happened, I wouldn't have met the wonderful people who have helped me on this journey, and my life is richer with those people in it. You also learn what real friends are, and you get the chance to become a better you!!!

29

Person with PNES, UK

My relationships with others have massively changed. I had worked through a lot of problems to build my confidence and become a strong woman who was independent and self-reliant. The day this condition started ruined all my hard work and stopped any positive part of me—the me that I had worked so hard to become, enjoying life properly.

After leaving my ex, the father of my children, who was a very abusive man, both physically and emotionally, I wanted to show my children that no one is allowed to hurt you, and that you must strive for more. I moved to a new house, lost weight, and changed careers—going from a very stable job to being self-employed and risking everything to "follow a dream." I was happy in my body, happy with who I was, and happy with who I knew I could be. I was in a great place, and non-epileptic attack disorder took it all.

Things slowly left me, and the scary thing was that I didn't see it happening. I knew I wasn't happy, and I knew I was cross, but now hearing what people have seen change over the last fourteen months is a very sad affair. I have seen things I didn't want to see in family members. I've seen how most of them didn't really care how my life was changing and that they are actually very selfish people, and I've felt hatred for them, which I never thought I would feel for my family. My dad was the only person who kept his heart and tried everything he could to help. I resent my mum more than I thought I could again. We had been on a tough journey after she left my dad; we didn't see each other for a number of years, and when we did, it was hard and there would be an atmosphere. I thought we were good after we made up again, but seeing how she has been through all of this has hurt. She really believes she's there for me, and that makes me cross. My now-wife, but at the time partner (we were still in the "getting to know each other" stage), had to give up her life to care for me when no one else would. I never thought that would ever happen. After all, you put your family first and would give it all up for them, but this never happened, not at all. This made me feel very alone and not worthy of their love; I didn't know why they didn't step in to help.

My friends were there from a distance, but they had their own lives and didn't really understand what was happening. I felt like I couldn't really talk about it, as when they asked questions, I couldn't even answer. I knew nothing about this illness and was ashamed of the parts I did understand. My wife was there every step of the way, and I really don't know how she could. I was horrible, even nasty, at times, and she knew that wasn't me and I didn't mean what I was saying. But it was hard work, and I owe her my life. I really don't know how others cope with non-epileptic attack disorder without someone strong to keep them focused.

The way people react is different. My wife is loving, caring, supportive, and knows what to say and do and when to do it, but no one else gets it. My mum makes fun of me, my dad gets upset, and friends panic. Strangers have been helpful, but they presume I have epilepsy. How on earth do you explain the contrary, and sometimes on a daily basis I have to explain the embarrassment of what it is. The doctors have ranged from blunt, confusing, and mean to only one doctor (and fortunately now mine) showing empathy and how she understood even just a little. I've heard lots and lots of stories of paramedics being extremely insensitive and downright mean, but thankfully I've not used the service, and so I have managed to skip the upsetting comments.

My independence vanished on day one, and being told by the first doctor we saw that I couldn't be left alone, especially with my children, felt like a knife. I was fiercely independent, especially after being controlled for so long. I had spent years alone with my children and having to make decisions and take the lead. It was tough not being "allowed" to do that anymore, and I suppose I tried to control as much as I could, though as it actually turned out, I just became mean and moody.

I lost my career, which was owning my own publishing company and being a full-time author, doing exactly what I loved and making a great living. I inevitably ended up being supported by the government, which made me feel terrible, and not at all what I had worked so hard for. I had only left my very stable job some five months previous, and this was a risky but worthwhile investment that I had made, and now I felt pointless. The way that the government makes you feel, like you're begging for money to feed your children, having to be interviewed and fill out mountains of reports and paperwork about how worthless you are to see if they can give you something to make ends meet. This is not what I fought for; this is not what I wanted.

I've been through a mile of emotions during the last 14 months. I've been frightened, scared, angry, hurt, and I've felt sadness and helplessness. Confusion has been mainly at the forefront of my mind throughout it all, with no professionals available for help or guidance. I've been referred for things to help, but still no appointments have been made. And even understanding how overstretched the hospital is, it doesn't help with the reality of day-to-day life, and the daily struggles we face dealing with this cruel illness.

I do understand non-epileptic attack disorder a little better now, and I suppose it's after coming to terms with my past. Having lived the traumas firsthand is bad enough without having to relive it with flashbacks and more with this illness. The idea that any professional has that a patient is "making it up" or "putting it on" breaks my heart when I'm swamped with nightmares and flashbacks taking me back to twenty-three years of hell that I can no longer forget. I now see certain triggers and find ways to deal with things before they can cause a seizure, but this is not always possible, and I live my life just waiting for the next one to usually ruin a great day.

I am lucky enough to have a wife who helps me to carry on with building great memories, even if there's lots of bad ones thrown in there. We now try to make extra good ones, to counteract the bad. We're a great team and manage this illness well. It's such a shame the illness is part of it, but we will fight on with the hope that one day it will go, and we have the knowledge we can get through anything.

30

Partner of Person with PNES, UK

Our relationship began in no extraordinary way; we found that we loved spending time together and very quickly found it difficult to be apart. We had the stress that this was a same-sex relationship, which was completely new to my partner, and although I knew I was gay, I had never had a serious relationship with a woman. We were always off on some adventure. She was extremely fit and had lost a huge amount of weight following a long period in an abusive relationship. I too had experienced a very difficult few years through ill health and my son's disability, but we found ourselves to be in a really happy place. In March, my partner and I had done a 23.5-mile hike just for fun. This was a big challenge for me, and I struggled fitness-wise. My partner, on the other hand, could have ploughed on for days without stopping. She gave me the push I needed to get fitter, and we both signed up to do an organized three-peaks challenge [a mountain hiking event in the UK] for a national charity in May. My partner was teaching regular Zumba dance workout classes, which I loved to attend, and was writing and publishing her much-loved series of children's books. She was fast becoming someone I both loved and admired, and who showed me that life could be good again. On top of all these things, she was an excellent mother to her two young children. They came before anything, and she loved to include them in almost every aspect of her life. At this point, we were taking the relationship at a nice steady pace.

In May, we had been together for around five months and were getting ever closer. We had begun to notice that she seemed to be having regular fainting spells. We found them amusing at first as it usually happened when she blew her nose or anything else involving a similar pressure. We went off to do a hike and soon realized that there was more to it. Unlike our previous trip, she was quickly tiring and seemed to be lacking in her usual boundless energy. The following week, she spoke to her general practitioner about the increasing fainting spells as it had now happened while she was driving, and the general practitioner asked her to come in immediately to have a few tests, including a blood test. While having her blood taken, she suffered her first full seizure. I was scared to see her this way. I took her home, and we were both very concerned. The coming weeks brought several more seizures, and I was asked by the general practitioner if I would stay with her. We had many appointments, for MRI, CT , more blood tests, and neurology. It was a really scary time for many reasons. We had been trying to take the relationship at a slower pace, and I was suddenly in the house all the time with my son, who had not spent much time there and due to his autism and other special needs was struggling to adjust. Our lives changed rather drastically overnight. My partner didn't know what was happening to her body, and I didn't really know what I was supposed to do about it. I wanted desperately to give her the space and time we had given each other previously; I knew that she was battling emotionally with the loss of independence and the need to parent her children alone, as she had done for a long time. I too wanted time with my son, if only to try and help him to understand what was happening. This was too difficult to do; her seizures were coming thick and fast and were often very long and violent, followed by long periods of confusion and exhaustion. Also, as a seizure was approaching, she would often become verbally combative and would not be able to listen to reason, so she would still get into a bath and then, if she were to go onto a full seizure, I was scared that she would cause herself serious harm or worse, and I didn't see how I could leave her knowing this was the case.

As much as the children seemed to be very understanding, they were too young to be able to deal with or cope with the events as they happened. I felt a little isolated as my friends often didn't seem to understand why I canceled plans with them. She was so distraught that she had lost so much of herself and that I was always there (in her eyes) as a "babysitter" that she seemed very withdrawn and annoyed a lot of the time. Neither of us really understood what was happening and had no real choice but to go along with it.

In July, my partner had a big seizure, which resulted in her being hospitalized for nine days. She had several seizures while in the hospital, and although we were given several possibilities as to what it could be, there were no real answers. I could see her becoming more and more withdrawn, and it was distressing to see. I loved her so intensely that I couldn't bear to see her in this way. I knew that other than being there, there was little I could do. I was extremely tired and emotional, and I knew that my partner withdrawing was not a good thing, and it scared me as I didn't want to lose our relationship because of this evil illness.

Through it all, we reassured one another and remained very much in the place of love that we had managed to build, but it felt different and uncertain. After leaving the hospital, we went to see a neurologist. He was very straight-talking and emotionless. We had gone to discuss the results of all the tests done while in the hospital. He bluntly said that he felt my partner had non-epileptic attack disorder and gave her a form to inform the Driver and Vehicle Licensing Agency of her illness. I was really worried as I knew that my partner considered this to be a form of mental illness, on par with the kind of illnesses that she would have made up herself. Neither of us at this point, like the illness and its origins, had been properly investigated, and all I knew was that my bright and bubbly, energized girlfriend was disappearing in front of my eyes. I wanted nothing more than to see the giddy and funny person that I fell in love with. I knew she was in there, but all I could see was an extremely scared and vulnerable person. She looked so alone and walked away from the appointment angry and confused. I rang the neurologist's secretary, who agreed to make an appointment to see another doctor, but it would be a little while before we would be able to. She also had a small cyst on her brain, and a repeat MRI test was arranged for the September. My partner was placed on a medication for the intense and painful headaches she was suffering, which she reacted badly to. It completely altered her mood, and she couldn't bear to be around people, including myself and the children. She didn't only seem to not love or want me around, but pretty much anyone. This again was distressing. It was difficult to explain her mood to the children, and as it was the school holidays, they were always around. I could see that their noise and persistent questioning of everyday things and their general playing was causing her to have more seizures. The noise and distraction was making it extremely hard for her. I knew that she was struggling with my son being around, and I knew he could feel this, which felt really tough. They didn't seem to understand that I couldn't split myself in four different ways, and I never quite figured out how to manage this, other than giving the children jobs when she had a seizure. I would send one for a glass of water, one for a blanket, and the other would fetch a pillow. Sometimes this would work, and other times it wouldn't. One time, my partner was about to fall off the sofa while fitting, the youngest child ran out of the house and hid across the road, and the middle child began to scream and shout because she wasn't getting what she wanted. This compounded the impact of the seizure as she would seize for longer periods if there were loud noises. Also, her extreme confusion when she came out of the seizure made her behave more in the manner of a small child, and she was not really safe to be alone. She would also cry and sob if I left the room; it was a very frightening time for her. I could see that clearly, but I just didn't know how I was meant to manage everybody's needs, and I was sorely disappointed yet not surprised at her family's lack of support with anything. Her father had recently been diagnosed with terminal cancer, yet he was the only person in her family who ever really tried to support us and at least acknowledge what a difficult time it was. I loved my partner and all three children very deeply, and I knew we could get through this. But I never really figured out how I could make it better, and the longer she was on the medication, the more I felt she resented my presence. I knew this for a fact as she was happy to tell me. She didn't like me to talk much and was fairly uninterested in most conversation.

The seizures were extremely intense and regular right through the summer. I wanted to give her the space we both needed, but her desperately more so, but after taking my son on a short holiday, I realized that there was not the appropriate support available if I wasn't there so I decided to stay. It wasn't an easy decision for either of us as we both needed the room to process everything that had happened in such a short time. We had both had so much to deal with, it felt nearly impossible to take it all in. I never saw myself as a carer, and I never would. I was there because I loved her and the children, I didn't feel the children should take that responsibility, and I didn't like the way other people "attempted" to care for her. Other than my son, I was willing to lose anything to be there for her. I shed a lot of tears, both privately and occasionally a little more publically, but not intentionally. As I had suffered a large mental breakdown some years before, I knew people were worried, and it was hard to have to keep answering their questions about a topic I find difficult at the best of times, especially when I knew that I wasn't suffering in that way. Yes, I was sad, but I did not feel anything like I did at that time.

At the beginning of September, she decided to stop taking the medication and regain some control over her life. It was like a real light-bulb moment; she woke up the following morning and told me with the "old her" sparkly eyes that she loved me. I wanted to cry; I had not heard those words, other than during her confusion following a seizure, for some time. At that moment, I knew that the world wouldn't be right overnight, and I was skeptical at this time as to how long this would last, but it really was truly a wonderful feeling.

September was good. There were still lots of seizures and uncertainties, but we felt like the formidable team that we had become early on, all over again. In the early days of October, she went with her mum to see her consultant; I was unable to go as I had a commitment with my son. We had felt quite positive about this appointment as we had been told to record all seizures and all other symptoms because the doctor did not feel that non-epileptic attack disorder should be diagnosed so quickly. We felt that someone was finally going to take the problem seriously. We had frequently found that doctors were interested while they thought it was epilepsy, but soon lost interest once there was no confirmation of this. Secondary symptoms were not being acknowledged, and the general practitioner quickly dismissed us out of hand. This was her chance to be taken seriously in our eyes. I was really upset that I was unable to attend as I had spent months painstakingly recording every symptom, seizure, and other thing affecting her health that were connected. I was also very nervous as we had been discussing moving in together properly, which had been a difficult topic as we had kind of been forced into it earlier than we would have naturally done it, but after several conversations, we agreed we would. I had not spent any real time in my own home for several weeks and felt very nervous about going back there as I had got into a new routine, had adjusted all my son's routines, and was worried what the impact on all of us returning to how things were before would be. Also, as the seizures were still happening, I wasn't sure how this would work, although we both agreed that even had it been for one night, me going home would have been nice, just to see that we missed each other.

I was nervous because of the reaction following my partner's previous appointment, and I didn't want us taking a step back. The consultant was rather unpleasant to her, and she left with no real answers other than to be told there would be another EEG done and an appointment to follow. I knew quickly that she was upset with this appointment, but she had that feeling about her that showed me she wasn't going back to that dark place. Everything was extremely tricky, and nothing seemed to be able to happen without a fight, but we were learning to live the best we could with the condition (whatever it was).

At the end of the month, she took me to a beautiful spa for the night as a birthday present. It felt wonderful to have that time with her by myself. We were so connected, and all I felt was love, and it was made even better by her proposing in the most wonderful way. It didn't matter what had gone on before; just knowing that regardless of any previous struggles she had faced, and whatever we were going through at the time, she wanted to marry me, it felt amazing. I had known for a very long time that I would marry her in a heartbeat.

It has been an extremely emotional and frustrating year, constantly seeing doctors who seem extremely unhelpful though interested, at least until they don't understand the condition. Trying to maintain family life with two children with additional needs, a third with emotional needs, and their age making it hard for them to fully understand why they shouldn't behave in a certain way, and not one professional understanding this. Trying to maintain what you know is the most wonderful relationship ever when you are tired and emotional and trying to keep so many balls in the air that you don't know which one will drop first. I have never been more scared than I have in this past year, scared that I will lose it all in a heartbeat, scared that she wouldn't make it. There was so much to lose and come back from if I lost her, either to illness or her feeling that she had to walk away. We have been extremely lucky, we have an incredible bond and we make the best team, and we know that we can weather any storm. We know that this could have destroyed our relationship with it starting so early on, and that hurts to my soul. I know that I have her and there will never be an event that ever makes me think that I don't want to be here. I can take the rough times, but this illness is evil and needs to be better understood and treated.

There needs to be better support for families like ours—we all have our burnout point. We are both extremely tired all the time, and we cry more than I ever have in my life. I like to think that one day the seizures will stop, but right now we don't know if or when that will be, and we don't know what the lasting effects on her health will be. Her memory is badly affected, and that causes her a lot of distress and upset—it's certainly frustrating for us both. We are young, our children are young and we want to live our lives to the full. Most days I'm good, other days I have a wobble, but we have each other. If there was more specific and available support, I think there would be less wobbly days.

31

Person with PNES, UK

I'm sick of never being able to get involved with anything, like stuff with my kids and family.

I've had seizures where I woke up not sure where I am or even remember who is with me.

I have always worked all of my life; I ran a very successful garage in a workshop. I can't even write neatly now.

My thoughts feel mushy, like I'm not sure what is real and what I dreamed. If I concentrate, I get pains in my head. I don't get blurred vision; it is more like I get more vision.

When I feel myself going mushy, as I call it, I can't make out conversations; they like all jumble together. I hear people who are there, I can sometimes see my wife or someone talking to me, but their words don't follow their mouths. It's like a strange dream world.

My biggest frustration is when I feel okay, I feel normal and like I could do anything. Then I try to do something like gardening, and I get mushy when I get involved. It's like I'm okay if I don't think, but I can't do that.

I feel angry that I am physically fit, but that I can't do anything safely.

I have always financially supported my children, but now I find it hard to support my wife and myself. Work is available for me, and I try to work, but within two hours, I need to lay down. It's quite ridiculous to be honest.

I find psychotherapy very patronizing as I can see what they expect me to say next. I lucid dream every night; I often wish I could dream normally. When you are aware of all reality without blinkers on, the world is a very cruel place, so I find I try to always look for good in the world. It is true that ignorance is bliss.

I just need to learn that I'm in control of my mind, that's the hard part.

32

Person with Epilepsy and PNES, UK

My epilepsy and non-epileptic attack disorder has affected my life in so many different ways. I have lost my job, driving, confidence, self-esteem, family, and friends.

I've been treated like **** at hospitals because of the dual diagnosis of epilepsy and non-epileptic attack disorder. I have been treated like I'm a fake, an attention-seeking person.

I've been laughed at and made fun of.

I've also met friends with the same condition who understand better than anyone else.

Every day, it raises its nasty head.

33

Person with PNES, the Netherlands

I am actually very embarrassed to basically sum up how my pseudoseizures have affected me in all sorts of ways. Although I try to keep things light and positive toward my friends, it has been quite difficult.

Where to start? I suppose—by now—it is safe to say that it has ruined me, basically. Having a seizure every one to two or two-and-a-half hours does not leave much room for anything else. I do not feel them coming, so that is not helping. It has been about six years now since I found out I have it. Since then, I have lost my job in children's day care (completely understandable, of course), which was my absolute passion. I have been on disability ever since and have been marked one hundred percent unable for work. The frequency of my seizures has become worse over the years. It is very rough physically too. Because of the fact that I barely sleep, pulling myself back up after each one is tough. Adding to it, I have cramped hands into fists, my right side is always stiff, muscles in my entire body are always cramped, walking is difficult, my energy is very low, my jaw is locked so I am on liquid food, my back is very painful all the time, and I have trouble swallowing (I throw up a lot, so I lost a lot of weight, too). In the beginning—when I was averaging six to eight seizures—it was not as bad as it is now. I could go out and visit friends every now and then.

I received treatment at a specialized clinic for epilepsy and pseudoepilepsy (and also trauma therapy for post-traumatic stress disorder), to no avail. After that specific department had to close and everyone was forwarded to mental health care, it was soon obvious that they could not help me either and lacked the knowledge. Nothing helped. What was I doing wrong? The inpatient program was changed into outpatient six weeks after I got there and lasted till the end of 2012. Since then, I have been referred to many mental health care places; for one center, I was refused after an intake meeting because it was "too complicated." That is how it has been up to now. I cannot seem to improve, nothing works, I get worse and worse, and nobody seems to be able or willing to take a chance on helping me.

I am incredibly mad at myself for not being able to overcome this myself, and even more for being like this in the first place. You are such a weakling! Useless, pathetic, loads of people have had bad experiences and they manage fine! You are worthless! You cost a lot of money yet contribute nothing to society! Just pull yourself together! No one you met in 2011 at the specialized clinic has seizures any more except you! Loser! Just some of my thoughts. Obviously not helping, but there nonetheless.

I am always at home or on my balcony smoking a cigarette. My body just does not work with me, and if I am out, I cannot walk too long. It is so painful and costs so much energy. Besides, people staring at you for walking funny or if I have a mark or wound on my face (I often do) is not fun. If I have a seizure, I am scared what people will do, and above all, I do not want an ambulance to take me to the Emergency Room. They cannot help me anyway, and it is so much fuss. Once people find out from reading your file or something that you have pseudo (or "fake") seizures, you can instantly sense a change in their behavior and how people talk to you. Awful.

I do not see my friends more than once or twice a year. I talk to them on the phone a lot, though; they are great. I think it is better this way for I am enough of a burden without them actually seeing me decline. I do not want them to feel bad. And I honestly do not want to be seen. By anyone. Not even them. I do feel very bad about it, though. The three of them who live in my town all have full-time or part-time jobs and children now, so they are busy enough as it is. One of them was very honest and said it would be too much of a burden on the kids to see me. I understand and agree completely, but it still makes me feel bad and guilty for being such an awful friend. Well, I am not even a friend in my opinion. I am nothing. I am not a part of anyone's life, absolutely useless, and have next to no hope left of ever getting better.

The physical things are not taken seriously by my general practitioner—in my experience—because of the psychogenic non-epileptic seizures and post-traumatic stress disorder labels: "It is just tension," "Just talk to the psychiatrist." You feel so lost, misunderstood, unheard, and utterly worthless. Even though I get up after every seizure and stand and walk it off, I sometimes think lately, why even bother? In an hour or two, it will be the same again. But then I think, stop feeling sorry for yourself, you #$$*.

Although I also have the post-traumatic stress disorder label, and I have had therapy for that too, I still think the actual seizures are the worst because they are disabling. I just wish things were different and that I could fix this somehow. I do not even think about the bad experiences in the past or anything. I just think, get up again and walk it off. Every day. Again and again. Pathetic story right? Pathetic person . . .

34

Person with PNES, UK

I end up having a seizure because I get really stressed over things. Thank God when people don't see me have a seizure. I only like my family to be around me. I get panicky if anyone else sees.

At bed time, I hate it: it is something about going to sleep that I hate. Sometimes I have stupid nightmares about my family members dying and about their funerals. It's horrible. I always listen to music before I sleep. It helps me to relax. It makes it easier to fall asleep.

In the mornings, I often have a seizure. My mum always checks up on me, just in case I feel like I am going to have, or if I have had, a seizure because I don't like to be on my own when coming around from one. Sometimes I am fed up and stressed for no reason; I think I am just fed up of being me! I do the same thing every day; my life can be boring! I want to be better, go out, get a job, have a life . . . but no! I always get told, "I'll get better." Two years later, I'm still like this, having seizures every day.

I try watching films to cheer myself up, I listen to music, do my color therapy book—but still nothing. It is when my mum talks to me about why I am stressed, it seems to help. I suppose talking about it always does make it better for a while.

I am currently doing a thirty-day chronic illness challenge; every day is a new question that I have to answer about my illness. I am on day 20; it is a question about meeting others with some illness. I've spoken to them but not met them. It helps to talk to others that are in the same situation; it makes me understand better that I'm not alone with how I feel.

When my eyes start to flicker, I know that I am going into a seizure. My eyes are my first sign (normally). Then my hands tingle, then I get a weird sensation in my head as if the room is spinning, then I don't remember anything else. The next thing I'm aware of is I am coming round not being able to breathe, coughing, looking around to see who's there. I have to lay there for about an hour for my head to stop pounding and for me to get focused. Every time I have a seizure, I always feel like rubbish afterward, another one added to the list. It's meant to be stopping, why isn't it all stopping? There is not a single day since April 10, 2014, that I haven't had a seizure.

I haven't been swimming in ages because I have to go with two people at least who can get me out quickly and safely if I have a seizure so I don't injure myself or worse. The joys of being normal. Hopefully, one day, I will get back to my normal self where I don't have to worry about having a seizure.

I don't always like meeting new people. I have bad anxiety issues. I've had cognitive behavioral therapy for it, which helps a lot.

I always have off days, but I do manage to pick myself up again.

35

Person with PNES, UK

My condition started off very severe. I was having over twenty seizures a day, and I was unable to function and live a "normal" life, whatever that is. I had treatment with neuropsychology, and all was good. I was seizure free for six months, but then I started work—you know, everyday normal things that people do. My disability living allowance was coming to an end; one of us had to work. I was going stir crazy and so decided it would be me; problem is, my seizures restarted. At first, I thought I was just in the wrong job (high-stress job working in a prison maybe wasn't the best career choice for someone who can't process stress correctly). Now I'm still in a stressful role working with medical records in a hospital. My seizures haven't gone away; they affect everything; they are frustrating, annoying, stressful in themselves; and I feel like I am a burden at work as everyone is currently walking on eggshells because they know that if I get too stressed and upset, then I'm likely to have a seizure.

The thing is, it is hard to explain the cause. It is also hard to explain the feelings before them, the "spacey feeling," that's the only way I can think to describe them. But this isn't really understood by colleagues. I have found that I am quick to anger and quick to tears in the last few weeks, but that if I am crying (because I'm stressed or feeling like I am failing), then there is a very slim chance of me fitting. Knowing the warning signs is key to getting through the day without one, but sometimes they sneak up on you and you have no or very little warning. Occupational health has deemed it unsafe for me to work alone, and so I now have to rely on colleagues to get notes from areas where no one is around. It's frustrating as well as making me feel like I am not as good a team member.

Relationships are hard; my husband is still unsure of how much he can share with me if he is having a tough time through fear of tipping me over the edge. I used to disassociate, so I would become a younger version of myself. That was hard on him, and he is worried about me going back to the dark place of twenty seizures a day with no job and unable to go out alone. Work is hard because they see someone who isn't functioning "normally" and don't seem to understand that there are no magic pills, just the need to find ways to cope. Some days I can't get out of bed because I am cluster seizuring and the tiredness from them is all consuming. I don't feel normal and feel I have to justify that I am coping okay when people ask and don't understand that a few a month, or even one a week, is so much better than I once was and if that is all I have to deal with I will take it gladly.

I feel that the doctor's and therapist's view of normal and coping, and the views of employers and the outside world, are mismatched, whereas my neuropsychologist was happy to discharge me having few, but manageable, seizures as being able to cope and no longer needing treatment. The outside world and employers especially don't see this as a breakthrough or as something that is correct. The way they see it, if you are still having seizures, then you need pills or you need more treatment. But my treatment was complete. I dealt with the big traumatic events. I can talk about them without going into a seizure or blind panic. I feel that those doors have been well and truly closed, but it's now the everyday stress that keeps my condition going. The stress and worry of holding a job down, of feeling like less of a team member because my now-deemed disability stops me from doing all the tasks that they can, of feeling like a failure if I have a bad day and can't go into work because I know that's one sickness period and that ultimately, if I have too many bad weeks, I could lose my job, which would mean financial worries for the family—I am the sole money earner, and although I am happy to be supporting my husband, who is wanting to become a counselor and is currently in training, it's a big burden for someone who can only hold so much stress at once. I feel bad when I have a seizure around my little boy for fear of scaring him, but so far, he seems used to them and deals with it well—even holding my head until I come round. I am now engaging with a life coach to see if learning some stress management techniques can help to tame the seizures so they do not affect my work life.

So what is it like living with non-epileptic seizures? Ultimately, it's rubbish, it's hard work, tiring, and I get very tired very quickly. I recently described my condition as being like a pressure cooker, and if you keep putting stuff in, eventually it goes pop (the way I had it described to me by someone). But I was challenged on this by someone that maybe instead of being a pressure cooker, maybe, just maybe, it was that I was like a glass of water that was nearly empty and in order to run, I needed to be full, so when I feel like my pot is full, maybe it's because my glass is empty and I need to take time for myself and to relax so that my glass or batteries are full and so my pot is bigger.

People react differently to my condition. Many people don't understand, and I resort to saying that it's like epilepsy, without the brain activity, and they get some idea of what it is like. I am currently having a hard time with describing it, not because I don't understand my condition, believe me I do (I have had it many years and am now coping with it and functioning as well as I can), but because I find that people are quick to judge the wrong way. We are considering adoption, and so I am going to have to go through the ins and outs of my condition with social workers. I am not sure how to approach it. Work colleagues are now getting used to my seizures and no longer panic, which helps me as it means the episodes are shorter and I can get back to work quicker. It has taken a few seizures for them to re-alize that I do not need to go to the hospital when I have one and that I can continue with work and do not need to go home.

Final thoughts are that my self-confidence is low because of my condition and that relationships can be hard. I am coping, but maybe I am relying on coping too much and I need to get my ass into gear to start work on beating these once and for all. Hopefully, that will happen over the next few weeks with the new stress man-agement coaching.

36

Person with PNES, UK

If you have to cry, scream, or shout, then do so, but then also write.

For a little while I find it is best to not use social networks, just so I can focus on my mental and physical heath. You do need to give yourself some slack and credit, and don't be so hard on yourself. We all start off not understanding why we have seizures. It doesn't make you a weak individual at all because seizures occur; it means that you have reached the breaking point and your mind cannot withstand it anymore.

Take each day as it comes, try to come to terms with what you have been through, but slowly. It's a process that shouldn't be rushed. Past traumas and events could be the cause behind your seizures; our mind is a powerful device that can subdue your conscious mind from the reminder of these events by causing seizures. It does that because you are not ready to face what it is, and the pain behind it could be more horrific then the actual seizure itself.

You need to find out your triggers so that you can prevent a seizure from occurring; you need to tune your inner self so that you know what your subconscious mind is trying to tell you. I found psychotherapy sessions very useful. I was able to fully see hidden things like thoughts and feelings that were once upon a time unseen. For example, I thought that I had forgiven my ex-partner for being physically abusive, but in truth, I hadn't and will never be able to forgive him for causing the miscarriage of my daughter, something that I pushed aside and never came to terms with until the day that I was told I was infertile and not capable of having more of my own children.

Just know that you are not alone. It's fine to be scared; I was scared too. Grasp hold of good memories, keep them close, and use them as a healing device, use them to help heal yourself. Face things straight away, and don't brush anything aside. Express every emotion, including anger, so that the healing process can begin. You can come out a stronger and wiser you. You have overcome challenges, traumas; you have battled against stuff that usually defeats the majority of people. It shows that you have amazing strength and the willpower to carry on.

Have faith in yourself; don't let these traumas diminish your faith in any way. The more upsets that you go through, the stronger your faith in yourself should become.

Don't let others pull you down because they don't understand exactly what you are going through. Surround yourself with supportive friends and family; I know it can be very difficult to stand on your own. Sometimes people only understand if they have gone through it themselves or seen someone else close to them go through it.

At times you may stumble, but that's okay—don't let these stumbles defeat you. You'll eventually get back up and carry on. Let friends and family aid you if they are willing to help you.

Try not to dwell on the past. You can choose to sit in perpetual sadness, immobilized by the gravity of your loss or pain, or you can choose to rise from it.

Take the lessons that are being taught; leave behind the heartache and pain. Live your todays while drafting your tomorrows.

End this chapter, and go write yourself a new one.

37

Person with Epilepsy and PNES, UK

I had my first non-epileptic seizure in June 2015. It was when I stopped taking my anti-epileptic medication, which may have acted as a barrier. However, I had had partial seizures for much longer but was unaware that there might be non-epileptic seizures too.

I have been seeing a psychologist for over a year now. We have been discussing grief and the loss of my father when I was aged six; I have struggled to cope with it for twenty-six years. When I have a non-epileptic seizure, I know that it is happening. My face feels paralyzed at one side, I struggle with my vision, yet I can hear perfectly. I just can't respond. It's like an out-of-body experience or a stroke; however, if I don't panic and try to stay calm, it normally passes quickly. Sometimes when I get worked up or stressed, it can also bring one on. How many seizures I have can depend on different things, for example, my monthly cycle, when I'm almost certain to have at least five small ones and two large seizures. Or if I'm stressed or upset, then I tend to have one. However, I think discussing grief helps because I had quite a lot of losses in my childhood. It came to the point where I wouldn't go to school for fear in case I lost my mum too, so I developed anxiety at a really young age (around seven or eight years). I think grief has played a large part because I hide most of my emotions about the loss of my father as it's not something that's easy to speak about. Maybe it was a buildup over the years with the fact that I take a high dose of an anti-epileptic drug that has caused it.

38

Mother of Person with Epilepsy
and PNES, UK

My daughter was diagnosed with epilepsy at the age of five. It was well controlled on an anti-epileptic drug. She would have the occasional absence seizures. At nine years old, my daughter had her first grand mal seizure. She didn't have another until she was eleven years old. In her teens, she started to have a few more grand mal and absence seizures; again, these were treated with more drugs. She went through normal times and did well in school, college, and went on to university. It was while she was at university that her health deteriorated; a water infection led to kidney infection. At this point, she was living in the halls [dorm rooms] but had to return home to live due to her health. She traveled daily to university. One evening while doing her work on her laptop, she went into status epilepticus and spent twelve days in the hospital; she was introduced to more drugs and was on a high regime. It took nearly a year for my daughter to be able to talk properly and put sentences together. On occasion, she still struggles with her speech to this day. The side effects of the medication were not good; she was constantly tired and feeling unwell, her hands would shake constantly. The grand mal seizures did lessen, but the absence seizures didn't.

We have seen numerous neurologists over the years; nobody mentioned the possibility of non-epileptic seizures until she was admitted to a hospital and seen by a specialist in non-epileptic attack disorder last year.

None of us had ever heard of these non-epileptic seizures before.

Two of the drugs that she was taking were interacting, so one of them was stopped. She started to experience more seizures. Some were grand mal/tonic-clonic, and the others were non-epileptic seizures, plus she experienced episodes of psychosis.

The non-epileptic seizures are very frightening, both for my daughter and for anyone who sees them. The first time I saw her in a non-epileptic seizure, I was very afraid of what was happening to her. I knew that it was different from her normal seizures as she didn't appear to be unconscious; only the top half of her body appeared to be in a seizure. Her mouth had drooped to one side (a bit like a stroke), her eyes were open wide and staring, they appeared to be full of terror, she was gasping, choking, thrusting her arms, and her head was jerking from side to side just like a grand mal/tonic-clonic. This non-epileptic seizure lasted about three or four minutes, and my daughter told me she knew it was happening and it felt like she was in a nightmare, and had no control of her body. She could see her body seize. She could hear everything I was saying and was trying to tell me to help her and that she was choking but couldn't get any words out.

My daughter comes round very quickly from these seizures; she doesn't have a headache nor is she sick after them like she is with a grand mal seizure. Another thing about these seizures is that she falls forward and not backward like she does in a grand mal seizure.

During one of these non-epileptic seizures, as my daughter fell forward she hit her chin on the kitchen worktop, and her teeth pierced through her lip, causing her great pain and discomfort. We went to the hospital to have it seen. Her experience at the hospital wasn't very caring. We try to avoid the Accident and Emergency Department as much as possible. On other occasions, she has banged her chin, her head, and chipped her front tooth.

Most of the absence seizures are very brief and proceeded by a noise; some have lasted no more than a few seconds. It appears that she has just frozen for a few seconds. She knows these absences are happening. Sometimes there can be quite a few in a day; other times just three or four in a week. Over the years, these have been diagnosed as partial, complex partial, or absence seizures. It is only since my daughter's referral to a specialist in non-epileptic attack disorder that light has been shed on the possibility that these are also non-epileptic seizures. I have noticed that some situations and stress can bring on these absence seizures. In the past, we have been treating these with medication, which seemed to stop them. We don't use this medication anymore as she is taking an anti-epileptic drug to help her seizures while another anti-epileptic drug is being reduced. It is difficult trying to reduce the anti-epileptic drug dosage on a regular basis as the grand mal seizures have increased dramatically in the last few months, which is making the reduction a very slow process.

I have noticed that before my daughter has any seizure of any type, she will appear anxious and agitated, which usually gives me an indication that she isn't feeling herself. Prior to a seizure, she will also tell me that she is not feeling well but can't describe what her symptoms are; the only description she can give is that she feels like she has had a seizure even though she hasn't.

My daughter is having psychological treatment to help her to deal with these non-epileptic seizures and learn how to try and control them when they occur. It is likely that the death of her father at a young age has had a deeper effect over the years than we have realized; this combined with many family losses and changes over the years, I believe, has all been too much for my daughter to handle emotionally.

It is very hard emotionally to see anyone suffer with this type of disability. The effect it has on the sufferer and the people around them is devastating. I am personally terrified when my daughter has a seizure; it breaks my heart to watch her, and the feeling of helplessness is awful. I am always terrified that she won't come out of the seizure or will go into status epilepticus again.

During the night, my sleep is very light. I am always listening and hoping that the bed alarm will go off if she has a seizure. On some occasions, this has failed, and my daughter has been face down in her pillow during a seizure, lacking oxygen and developing a petechial rash. This event has made her very nervous. The light has to stay on, and the family dog has to sleep in her bedroom (the dog is very good at alerting me when something is wrong). Sometimes I sleep in the same room as my daughter and sometimes in the same bed; mostly, I sleep in the bedroom next door to hers.

Life at present is very hard for her; she feels like she has lost a huge part of it, especially her independence and health. Her confidence has plummeted, she is afraid to be alone, but hates to feel what she describes as dependent.

My life is solely committed to my daughter's safety and welfare. I don't sleep very well, and my mind is always on alert. One small part of my mind is concentrating on what I am doing while the rest is listening out for unusual noises that will tell me something is wrong with her. Every minute of the day and night, my mind is on observation duty; it is very draining not be able to switch off. Seeing my daughter deteriorate and the change in her over the years is very hard to watch; one feels helpless and not being knowledgeable enough to understand exactly what is happening. I tend to research as many areas as I can to get any information that will increase my understanding of these seizures and ways that I can help my daughter to cope.

I have found that very few people, even in the medical profession, have ever heard of non-epileptic seizures, and I can quite easily understand from a visual point of view how closely these resemble epileptic seizures and how a diagnosis could be misinterpreted. My daughter's control of epilepsy over the last few years has not been fully achieved despite large amounts of different medications that have created other problems. In my mind, I now wonder how long she has been having non-epileptic seizures. Were the absence seizures that she has had throughout her life non-epileptic seizures that didn't respond to epilepsy drugs? These questions go through my mind constantly, and I wonder what the situation would be today if this is the case and she had been diagnosed years ago.

I have found that some friends and family have taken a step back from our lives. I find that my daughter is not included or invited to some events, just in case she isn't well. This makes her feel like she's a problem for some people, and it doesn't do her self-esteem any good at all. Some have taken more interest and try to help as much as possible; they also would like to know more about non-epileptic seizures.

I have noticed that some people talk over my daughter, and this intimidates her. It is usually due to the fact that it can take her some time to explain her feelings or get across what she wants to say as sometimes she is repetitive and slow in her speech; this may appear to others that she has learning difficulties. My daughter is an intelligent young lady and still spends time learning. It has only been since the status epilepticus that her speech has been affected in this way.

My daughter is unable to work or drive. Some days she is totally exhausted and will spend most the week sleeping. She doesn't have the energy to do much exercising, and this worries me, as does how it will affect her heart and circulation. Some days she is very depressed and nothing is right for her. She lacks male company; boyfriends in the past have not been able to cope with her epilepsy.

We have just been approved for continuing health care. This has taken a while to set up, although the local authority provided some care after my daughter had status epilepticus. This has been a great help to me and has enabled me some time to do things and rest. Going through the procedure of qualifying for this care has been very difficult for my daughter to handle. Most of the meetings left her feeling inadequate, disabled, and dependent. Everything she doesn't want to be. She has been emotionally upset after these meetings.

I think that the everyday things you take for granted are all of a sudden restricted when epilepsy and non-epileptic seizures are diagnosed in your family. Just popping out to the shop, keeping appointments, having a shower, making plans for holidays, etc. All these things along with many others are limited, and supervision for her needs must be arranged for me to just go out to the shops or walk our dog. Plans often change or are cancelled.

I am proud of my daughter and the way she strives to keep some normality in her life in any way she can.

I hope that my experience of my daughter's non-epileptic seizures is of some help to others. I think a forum of this would be a good help to anyone who is experiencing this.

39

Person with Epilepsy and PNES, UK

I had a really busy week this week. A week that was both mentally and physically very hard. However, no matter how hard the week was, I did it. I got through it! Monday started as a normal mundane day at work. I really didn't think I would have enough work to last the day, so I started to feel a little unenthusiastic about being at work. This feeling didn't last long at all. Things started to change, and I ended up having plenty to do. The rest of the day went relatively quickly, and it was soon time to go home. Once home, I needed to get my stuff ready for going away the next day. I felt a little nervous as my seizures had been particularly frequent the last three weeks and I was a little worried that I may have them while I was away. I got my stuff packed and then made dinner. As normal, I ate this with my husband on the sofa while watching television. We watched some television and I went to bed at about 9 p.m., read for half an hour, then went to sleep. Tuesday came, and it was time to get to the train station. My friend dropped me off, and I was about twenty minutes early for the train. I sat and listened to music until it arrived. The train journey was fine. I had a good book on the go, and it was nice just to sit and read for three hours. I had chosen to wear my shorts, so despite the warm weather I was very comfortable. When I reached the station, I recognized two people standing outside. They had organized a lift to the center, so I accompanied them. They were very chatty. I felt really tired after the train journey and found it quite difficult to add to the conversation.

Once we reached the center, we had food and the meeting started. I'm not used to sitting and listening, so after about an hour, I could feel myself becoming dissociative. I felt frustrated as these people were from head office and I didn't want them to see me like that. It had already been a massive struggle to get them to allow me back to normal duties. I didn't want them to question their decision. I'm really not sure if they noticed the vacant episodes that I had during the meeting; they didn't mention it, which was a relief.

The meeting finished, and it was time to go to the hotel. By this time, I felt really tired and didn't really contribute to the conversation in the car. We got to the hotel, and everyone was going to get changed before going to meet in the bar. Despite being tired, I agreed that I would also do this. God, I felt tired. However, being slightly silly [in the UK this is a figure of speech meaning to do something despite your best judgement], I went up to my room, got changed, and met them in the bar. I had a really good chat with a friend that lives abroad. She had been through a really rough time and had spent time in a psychiatric ward. She had been diagnosed with a mood disorder. We chatted about mindfulness and meditation, something we both try and practice on a regular basis. Talking to her spurred me into practicing it more frequently. We went and sat down for tea. I was sat between two people that were fairly difficult to speak to, although I did make an effort. I ate and chatted while waiting for dessert. All of a sudden, I didn't feel quite right, my speech slowed, and it became harder to move my eyes. In a wave, a vacant episode came over me, and all I could do was stare—I tried to get out but I was trapped. People started to notice and tried to talk to me, but I couldn't talk back to them. They wanted to help me back to my room, but I was worried that I wouldn't be able to walk properly. Eventually, by them asking questions and me nodding, they understood that I just needed to be left alone. God, it was frustrating. I just sat there willing it to pass. Then, as quickly as it came on, it went away, as if someone had opened the door to my prison cell. I ate my desert, then went up to my room while I could. I lay on the bed ready to read my book, but I was absolutely exhausted and couldn't keep my eyes open.

I was very tired the next morning. We left the hotel and went back to the center to finish the meeting. The second part of the meeting went by in a mixture of normality and vacant episodes. Eventually, it was time to catch the train home. The train journey home was very tiring. I had multiple vacant episodes, which led to slight convulsive movements on a couple of occasions. I managed to make all of my changes and made it home, although I was exhausted. I couldn't talk properly, and I was unable to walk properly. I had some tea and went to bed.

I woke up this morning feeling very tired. I had a pretty frustrating day yesterday, with one of the worst seizures I had ever had first thing in the morning. It wiped me out for the rest of the day, and I still didn't feel good when I woke up this morning. I made myself get out of bed and get showered. Trying not to be negative and trying not to dwell on how rubbish I felt was hard. I'm not sure you get used to struggling through your time at work. Every time, it feels like a massive uphill struggle, and at the end of it, all you have to show for it is that you managed to get through a day at work! I often think that if I struggled through that day, then this medical disorder would get better and I wouldn't have to go through it again. It would be much more motivational.

40

Person with PNES, the Netherlands

I have had non-epileptic seizures for many years. It all started when I was seventeen years old. I was just going to live on my own because it was terrible at home. The relationship between my mother and I was very bad. The seizures started out of the blue. Everyone thought that it was epilepsy, so the doctors gave me medication. Of course, the medicine didn't do what it was supposed to do, and the seizures kept coming. Rather serendipitously, there is a specialized epilepsy clinic in the town that I was living in. After a lot of admissions to the hospital, a neurologist sent me to the epilepsy clinic. After just one seizure, they knew that it was not epilepsy. It was a real shock to me; I had never heard of pseudoseizures before. It felt like they told me I was a faker. My first reaction was to run away from the clinic, that I didn't need help because it is just a mental illness. A few months later, I went back to the clinic and started a very difficult and intense therapy. It helped me a lot, but I was never seizure free.

Thinking about how it has affected my life, I'm now thirty-four years old, married, no kids and happy with three cats. The feeling that I was a faker is nowadays still present. Even my family and friends don't believe me that the seizures are part of a mental illness. I don't have many friends because I scare them with my seizures, and my colleagues don't know that I am sick. I have had many jobs, and when I told the manager that I have seizures, they always ended my contract, mostly instantly. Now I'm working and have never told them that I have seizures, and it is going well. Nowadays, I don't have many seizures. A good day rhythm for me is very important. I was unemployed for three years, and I developed depression and a spasm (the spasm is related to the non-epileptic seizures).

I tried every treatment there is. Psychiatrists, psychologists, neurologists, medications (anti-depressants, anti-epileptogenic), different hospitals, cognitive behavioral therapy, drama therapy, music therapy, you name it, I've tried it. Not every doctor has taken me seriously. Especially at Accident and Emergency

Departments, they have mistreated me. They don't take you seriously with mental illness.

My seizures are always the same; I am absent and start falling down and then have convulsions. During that time, I am completely unconscious. I do not respond to pain stimuli, my oxygen level drops, my blood pressure goes sky high, and my lactate level increases.

41

Person with PNES, UK

I have experienced non-epileptic seizures for twelve years. I was referred for cognitive behavioral therapy, but the counselor had never heard of non-epileptic seizures and it didn't feel particularly useful. I attended approximately five sessions and felt that it did nothing. In my first year of having them, I suffered between three and five a day for a couple of weeks, and then they would disappear, and then return in the same way. Now I only suffer with them if I've been really ill.

First and foremost, I have a huge issue with the name of this "illness." I feel like it's already setting us up to be misunderstood or not taken seriously. Non-epileptic seizures? What does that even mean? That's a truly terrible name. When you're only describing something by saying what it isn't, well that's not describing it at all. I don't use those words. I much prefer the term *dissociative seizures*. At least that way, it gives a tiny indication of what I go through. And what is it that I go through exactly? A feeling that I'm slowly ceasing to exist. Imagine for a moment that you can be turned off. That there's a button somewhere. But it's not instant. It's a slow process. Your whole sense of reality starts becoming less real. You can hear the voices of the people around you. But for some reason, your brain has suddenly forgotten how to respond. A chair isn't a chair anymore; in fact, you have no idea what it is. It feels like the ground is about to fall away, and yet you don't know where the ground is. It is scary. And yet you know the more you panic, the worse this is going to get. You can literally feel your brain and body going into fight or flight, but you don't know which is doing what. I've had different parts of my body go numb or tingle. I go all shaky, feel sick, and feel like I'm just going to collapse. Sometimes I don't know where I am or what's going on. Nothing makes sense. I even suffered with sleep paralysis during one horrific episode. I was suffering with seizures every day, three to five a day. But whenever I tried to sleep, I would fall into this state that was neither awake nor asleep. It was like I was hallucinating. It sounds crazy, but the Grim Reaper would be coming toward me and I would try to scream but no sound would come out. That was the worst experience. Worse than anything else I've experienced.

I've lost jobs because of it. I've woken up on the floor with my five-year-old daughter at the time sitting there looking frightened and just holding my hand. I was once thrown out of my daughter's school because of it. I was eight months pregnant, I could feel one coming on, I simply asked for some water, and they told me that I needed to leave. So I've been humiliated. I've had seizures while pregnant and feared for the life of my baby. I've had family think that I'm bringing them on because I used to suffer with anxiety, so therefore it was just simply something that I could control. It even made me wonder if I was bringing them on. After all, this wasn't epilepsy. So therefore it is I who's causing it, isn't it? But I have as much control over that as I do with the rash that appears on my chest when I'm nervous. My body has physical reactions that link directly to what I'm feeling. So yes, anxiety, nerves, and stress seem to be a trigger. But other triggers are flashing lights combined with loud club-type music. So that means nights out with my friends can't involve clubs. A huge trigger these days is if I've been unwell and haven't eaten or drank anything. I need to make sure I eat and drink. If I don't, I know it's going to cause problems. Which means if I get a stomach bug, I'm in big trouble.

I've had doctors look at me as though I'm making it up. I've spoken with several doctors who have never even heard of it. I should point out what my seizures look like to others. I have what look like absence seizures and grand mal seizures. So I either look like a zombie or my whole body is shaking very violently. I've had people try and pin me down. People have walked away and left me. And I've had others who have been sitting there holding my hand when I wake up. Some people have been wonderful, and others not so much. I've had the seizures at home on my own; I've had them when I've been on my own with my children. I've had them in supermarkets and shops. Ambulances have been called, and I refuse to go to hospital now because there's no point. I've never received any real help for this because no physical problem can be identified. I've fallen on glass tables, marble floors, and have been rushed into the hospital on those occasions because of worries about possible skull fractures. So when I've read that people with non-epileptic seizures aren't in any danger, I can't help but feel the seriousness of non-epileptic seizures is being seriously underestimated.

I can't tell you the amount of times either that I've wished this was epilepsy. Now I'm sure people who suffer with epilepsy would tell you I wouldn't want that. But at least it would have a name and people would understand it. I might have been given some form of medication to help control it. After all, I have what looks like epilepsy, I suffer with seizures, but there seems to be no real explanation for it. Some even seem to think that it's all in my mind. Well if it is, could someone tell my mind to get rid of it please, because it's kind of been ruining my life. The seizures have become less and less, though, so for that, I'm grateful. And I do have a couple of techniques that I learned when looking it up on the internet. Try and focus. I focus on a piece of material, I try and think about how it feels, what it looks like, just one simple thing, and just concentrate on it. If I can hold onto that then maybe I can hold onto reality; maybe I won't cease to exist. Maybe my mind won't "switch off." And someone talking calmly and quietly to me always helps, and strangely enough, if they make jokes, that helps too. I think it's the panic and fear that I'm feeling that seem to worsen everything. It's like how if you're stressed, it can cause a headache. There's nothing physically wrong, but the stress still causes an unwanted response. Same with this. These days, if I get a stomach bug, my body becomes weak, I will feel dizzy, my blood pressure drops, I will feel panic, I will feel anxious and scared and experience the warning sign, which is that feeling of dissociation from everything. And then that's when the seizures happen. But if someone is there talking to me, holding my hand, joking (which I know is hard, but it's my husband who does this and it does work!), then seizures don't always happen. It's as though my mind is fighting to hold on. And I'm fighting my own body to not go into the seizure.

It's incredibly difficult to explain. But we need to try. We need to get it out there that these types of seizures are real. They're as real as epilepsy. They're scary. There isn't an easy way to control them. Cognitive behavioral therapy probably would be a good route to go down, if only therapists have heard of them. It has been ten years since I sought help; I hit so many brick walls, I gave up. Perhaps there is medication out there for them now. I hope so. We need two things: a way to help control them and understanding. Maybe that way we can go back to living more "normal" lives.

42

Mother Whose Daughter Had PNES, UK

Our daughter was diagnosed with non-epileptic seizures between the ages of about twelve and eighteen years. This diagnosis followed various tests and scans, including a sleep-deprived EEG test and a referral to a children's hospital, where we saw a consultant who actually told us that these incidents could possibly be caused by hormonal changes in her body and would hopefully disappear in time. This seems to have been proved to be the case. At the time, however, we had never heard of such a condition, and could find very little information on it that would help our particular circumstances. We therefore felt extremely isolated in dealing with these "events" when they occurred, and it was only when our general practitioner eventually referred us to a psychiatrist that we felt we had any sort of support. We had regular, family orientated appointments with him whereby my husband, daughter, and myself would all sit down for a detailed chat about various experiences that had happened throughout our daughter's childhood. These included her grandma going through cancer treatment and eventually passing away, and also seeing a very dearly loved pet cat get killed outright by a hit-and-run driver. Our understanding at the time was that these negative experiences could in some way have contributed to the seizures that she was suffering from, and indeed, these seizures seemed to be a sort of cutoff mechanism, which helped her block out negative thoughts. This, however, seemed a bit of a paradox as we began to find that on occasions, they actually seemed to exaggerate her negative thinking with visual hallucinations.

During her seizures, she would "blank out" completely and was totally unaware of where she was or whom she was with. There were many instances where I was called out of my job as a teacher to go to her aid, either at school or indeed to various locations that she had been found in. It was a constant worry for us, on a day-to-day basis, not knowing if or when the next seizure would happen. Another symptom of these seizures was that sometimes when she blanked out, she would draw, write, or even scribble VERY negative pictures or writing. These included compulsive writing of the same phrase over and over: " Me, you, and your killer." During some of her seizures, she would have visual hallucinations about people being killed, and the manner in which these "murders" took place. She suffered severe panic attacks on "coming round," and often felt that there was something tight around her throat. Also, following an attack, she would complain of a headache and feel very tired. I have got many letters from school regarding incidents that happened. I have also got examples of writing that she did while having a seizure. Worryingly, there were several occasions when she would lose her memory following a seizure. One time, she was admitted to the hospital as she was unable to recite the alphabet in the correct order, and also the days of the week and months of the year. Another time, she couldn't remember who her brothers were on a family portrait that we had on the wall.

Obviously, I can't begin to tell you how concerned we were because, apart from the psychiatrist, we felt that we had nowhere to turn for help and felt completely isolated, as though we were the only family that had ever gone through something so distressing. Eventually, the psychiatrist referred our daughter to a hospital day unit, where she learned to practice skills that helped her to cope with her anxiety and panic attacks, and also the inevitable bullying that she had to deal with on a daily basis at school. Thankfully, after about six years of suffering these seizures, they gradually became less and less frequent, and I am happy to report that around the age of eighteen, she finally became symptom free, apart from it leaving her with memory problems. This must give hope to a lot of people who believe that they are stuck with similar symptoms for life—there can be light at the end of the tunnel. I would like our daughter to contribute to this book, giving her version of events; however, I am not prepared to let her visit this dark time in her life for fear of a re-surgence of the symptoms. She is now happily married, and in a very good place in her life, and we don't want anything to affect that happiness.

43

Person with PNES, USA

My condition has been really rough for my family and me. Before I was diagnosed, it scared everyone in my family because when I have a seizure, I black out and have no idea what is going on and wake up sometimes groggy and really weak, not knowing who or where I am. I can see what it has done to my family, especially my wife—just seeing the look on her face when she wants to help but just doesn't know what to do.

Over the last three years, I have lost my home, my job, and my freedom. A lot of the times, I feel totally worthless to everyone and myself. If I do too much during the day, I go into seizures and am out most of the day. My wife and I have been together for nineteen years, and most of it, she hasn't needed to work because I was making enough to support our family and us. Now I can't work because of my seizures, and I feel like a failure to my family. Even though I have been told not to worry about it by my family and friends, it's hard not to when you go from the breadwinner of the family to someone who can't support himself.

Even though I have great support from my family, it's really hard for me to handle all of this. Trying to find a doctor I can talk to about this or a therapist I can go to has been a total pain. I've gone through three counselors since this all started, and now I am without one again. There just isn't the support that I think I need. Just seeing what it does to my kids has been really hard, especially with my ten-year-old son. He wants to play soccer or baseball, and a lot of times I'm so out of it or really weak that I am unable to. The look on his face makes me feel like a worthless parent.

This condition seems to have taken my life away from me. I am trying things to work around the feeling and make things better, but it's really hard to do some-times. I used to go out all the time with friends and family, but now I'm afraid to because I'm scared of my seizures happening in front of people. I mean, what can I do? I want to go have fun. Go out to a ball game or walk along the beach with my family or go bike riding or drive again. But the seizures have been holding me back from doing any of that. I am at a loss and do not know what else to do. I don't like being in this funk of feeling helpless or worthless. At times, I feel like a burden to my whole family. I just wish there was a way to have it all go away and not have to worry about my condition anymore and get back to normal. I just need some help.

44

Person with Epilepsy and PNES, USA

May 3, 2013, was my very first one. I was with my boyfriend at the time in his home. We were being a little bit intimate when it started. It lasted about five minutes. My body began thrashing wildly, my head was jerking from left to right, and my limbs were hitting my body and the bed, I was completely out of control of my movements; however, I was completely conscious of him trying to talk to me and that he was watching me. He did not know what to do to help me, so he just stood there, watching, and helpless. Once I finally stopped shaking and flailing around on his bed, he tried to sit me up. I eventually sat up, but all the while, an arm would twitch, or a leg would jerk, or my head would shake. I was unable to speak because I kept stuttering or staring off or rolling my eyes. Each time I attempted to talk, only groans would come out or chattering of my teeth or biting my tongue, or even a sucking of some sort. Eventually, after putting some warm clothes on, very slowly, I could say short sentences and told him what I was feeling. My neck hurt from all the jerking back and forth, but other than that, I was simply exhausted. I had to urinate so I went to the bathroom. I could not. I came out of the restroom and asked for a sugary drink, thinking that perhaps it was an epileptic seizure and I needed some sugar in my system. He even took me outside for some fresh air. All the while, I was twitching and speaking oddly and staring off at nothing. I was unable to focus at all. Eventually, we went back into his bedroom, and we tried to watch a television show. He gave me some sleeping pills, hoping it would calm my body. I could not pay attention to the show because I'd end up staring off or shaking my head or jerking around. I was afraid to drive home and didn't know what to do, so I tried to lie down to sleep. All the while lying there twitching and jerking for about twenty minutes until I fell asleep (he stayed awake to watch me all night). I woke up a few hours later to find that I was back to normal. I went and was able to use the restroom at last. Went back to sleep when I was able to. No more twitching or anything.

The next day, I went home and told my family all that had happened. I was to see my sister's doctor the next day, and I rested all day in bed.

When I saw the doctor for the first time, I told her all about what had happened, and she immediately started me on a medication for epileptic seizures. I was supposed to start work at my new job that week, though, so she started me on a low dosage, hoping that the seizures would decrease. I had gotten the job offer a week before my first seizure. Perhaps this was a shock to my system, getting such a high-paying job. So strange, right? So what happened next? I had maybe two more seizures in the week before I sat down and saw the doctor. She told me the next time I had one to let her know. I did. The next Monday, after realizing that I was having an allergic reaction a few days after starting the medication, I presented with bumps underneath my skin under my ears and on my neck. I had a seizure in front of my parents and family at home, and they took me to the Emergency Room. The doctor decided to run a CT scan because the last time I was there, I'd had one due to a car accident that I had been in and they wanted to see if the two things were possibly related. They gave me a shot of the same medication I'd been on, and I was itchy all over my body, so they gave me a shot of an anti-histamine to stop my reaction. They decided that I'd need to go in for an MRI scan with dye and without (to see if something inside my body was causing the seizures) and also be hooked up to an EEG machine to test the electrical impulses and activity in my brain. So I was put in contact with someone local whom I could get these tests done with.

One major obstacle in my way with all of this doctor nonsense was that I was at the time uninsured. Luckily for me, I could sign up for emergency benefits due to these seizures coming out of nowhere and me being unemployed when it started. I immediately signed up before my first day of work and would have the benefits in just a few short weeks. Amazing what you find out from doctors these days! So I got into gear and got all my paperwork turned in in just a day. Now I just had to wait for the funds, or I could pay cash for the tests. I attempted to try to get the neurology tests started up by contacting a doctor friend of my doctor, and they basically turned me away. So my physician advised me to go to the medical center so they could admit me and run all the tests that I needed to have done. I informed my new employer and was off to get myself admitted to the hospital as soon as possible.

With my dad and sisters at my side, they helped me go through all the questions and such in order to be admitted to the medical center. This place was very quick with admitting me. Within two hours, I was on my way up to get my MRI test. Once done with this scary test full of loud noises and whirs, they brought me back to my little room so they could begin hooking me up to a twenty-four-hour EEG machine. The goal of my doctors? To capture me having a seizure with it so they could figure out the source of the seizures. All this talking to doctors was making me so nervous. I was such a shaken-up mess and so afraid. My sisters were coming and going to see me once I was admitted, and my boyfriend came to stay the night with me here and there when he wasn't at work. Such a sweet thing to do. He was so frightened for me, the poor thing; I will forever appreciate him for all that he did. Sticking by my side like that through it all. My family as well. All calling me and checking up on how things were going with the tests.

When my boyfriend had left for work the next day after being admitted, my dad took over babysitting me the second evening of being admitted. My dad was just talking to me, asking me how my day had been, when I began trying to tell him and my mind went blank and I started staring at him and my breathing stopped. The nurses had placed these giant cushions on the rails of my bed in case I had a seizure so I wouldn't harm myself. Good thing too! A seizure started, and I was hitting those cushions like crazy with my arms and my legs kicking, and my head hitting the cushions as well. Shaking back and forth like crazy. I could hear my dad yelling down the hallway that I was having a seizure to the nurses. Immediately, I could sense them all around me, trying to talk to me and communicate something to me to calm me down. Eventually, I stopped, and they told me to let them know that I was okay by moving an arm on my own. I did so and waved softly at them. I was exhausted and sure that I'd finally be able to sleep properly. An odd little fact: Once I had my initial seizure, each one following was anywhere from twenty seconds to a minute long. Nothing lasted as long as that first one. I think something clicked in my brain, though not sure what it was.

Now all I had to do was wait as patiently as possible for the test results from the video-EEG and the MRI test. I had to wait almost twenty-four hours for it all.

The team of physicians, including the main doctor on my case and the underlings that were learning from him, all entered my room the morning of the third day after being admitted into the medical center. What the doctor told me was a relief, but also a major concern to myself and my family.

The attending physician informed us that the MRI test they had taken proved to show no signs of any tumors or signs that anything in my body was producing the seizures. He then went on to tell us that the video-EEG test they took of me in order to record a seizure had shown that indeed there was no sign that any electrical misfires in my head were occurring, so what I had was not at all epilepsy. They decided to tell me that what was happening was referred to as "pseudoseizures," which in regular people talk means that they are psychological and that nothing was medically wrong with me. They told me that they would be sending a psychiatrist in to speak with me and evaluate me later that day. With that, they all exited the room.

I must admit that I was somewhat disappointed in the result. Not that I was disappointed I did not have epilepsy, but that there was no medication the doctors could offer to fix whatever was wrong with me. That no tumor was someplace in my body that could have been removed in order to make these seizures stop. That there was no "easy" solution to what was happening to me. Sending in a psychiatrist meant to me that this was going to take time and that there was indeed no simple solution to what was happening to me.

After waiting hours and hours for the psychiatrist to show up, she finally arrived around 2 p.m. that afternoon to begin her evaluation. She asked me if what I was going to discuss with her could be spoken about in front of my father, and when

I looked to my dad, I immediately said no (not because it had anything to do with him, but due to the fact that there were just some things that my dad did not know about me). She went ahead and asked him to leave the room until she was done speaking with me. He left slowly, unsure as to why I'd asked for this, but still prepared to allow the doctors some space.

She began by asking me if I had been in therapy before and if I had had any mental illness previously. I started out by explaining that I'd always had issues with anxiety since I could remember, and that in high school, I had my bouts of depression like other teens but a bit worse, I felt, since I was on some heavy medication for my acne, which really upset my mental state. I also explained that in the most recent few years, I'd began to have panic attacks as well, which I believe stemmed from some sexual abuse that had happened to me when I was in high school. However, more recently, in 2011, during the winter holidays, a family member's significant other had sexually assaulted me. What stemmed from that occurrence was the worst depression I had ever been through in my life. I would cry for an hour or more every day of 2012 for over six months. Only when I was encouraged by my best friend to start preparing for a five-kilometer run and started to have a healthy exercise routine did things start to improve drastically. I stopped crying for the most part unless I spoke about the assault from the previous year, or if flashbacks took over my mind as they tended to do. I had also gone through hallucinations and other things that upset me.

Upon hearing my stories and happenings in my life, the psychiatrist that evaluated me concluded that I had post-traumatic stress disorder mainly, and that my seizures most likely were related to that and called psychogenic non-epileptic seizures and so were psychologically produced. Along with post-traumatic stress disorder, I had a generalized anxiety disorder, depression, panic disorder, and a touch of obsessive-compulsive disorder. The list seemed to go on and on. She suggested that since I did not have medical insurance, I should seek a cognitive behavioral therapist to talk to and a regular psychiatrist that could regulate some medication with me and a schedule to follow and work on with my therapist.

She eventually left my hospital room and brought my dad back in. I told him what she'd told me, and he carefully did not ask too many questions. At the end of this, a nurse came in and began prepping my trip out of the hospital so that I could return home at last. The next week, I started at my new job; I held that job for almost a year. I also sought out a therapist to begin my healthy recovery. All through this time, the seizures continued on . . .

45

Person with PNES, Australia

I first started experiencing non-epileptic seizures three years ago. I thought these seizures were strange panic attacks as they are preceded by anxiety. During my seizures, my eyes roll in my head, and I lose control of my sight. I also shake and shudder throughout my body. I do not lose consciousness and can hear and understand what is happening around me. My seizures can last from one to eight hours and are very intrusive.

As I thought that I was having panic attacks. I saw a psychologist and did cognitive behavioral therapy for ten sessions, but I found this to be useless as my attacks didn't lessen. I struggled on for another two years with weekly seizures, including having them at work as well as at home. After having a seizure in the presence of my parents, they took me to the mental health crisis unit where I saw a psychiatrist. The psychiatrist insisted that I was having panic attacks despite my parents describing the strange eye rolling and shaking. I was prescribed an anti-depressant and told to see a psychologist for therapy. My sister, who had been in my company when I had a seizure, insisted that I seek a second opinion. I spoke to my doctor about my symptoms, and she was at a loss as to what to diagnose my condition as. I asked for a referral to a neurologist, and she agreed and said she would be very interested to hear what he says. I also went for an EEG and CT scan, and the results were sent to the neurologist. My appointment with the neurologist was excellent, and for the first time, I felt that I was receiving accurate information and a diagnosis. The neurologist said I was having non-epileptic seizures but wanted some further tests to rule out epilepsy. I was sent for a sleep-deprived EEG and an MRI. The results were clear, and I was referred to a neuropsychiatrist to treat non-epileptic seizures.

In the meantime, I had commenced seeing a clinical psychologist for anxiety and panic attacks. After I received the diagnosis of seizures, I spoke to the psychologist about this, and he told me that he had no training or experience treating seizures but was prepared to keep working with me. He commenced eye movement desensitization and reprocessing therapy with me, and we worked through a number of traumatic experiences that I had been through. I am currently still seeing this psychologist and continuing with the eye movement desensitization and reprocessing therapy, which is helping. At the moment, I am having one seizure a fortnight, which is an improvement from having three a week before I started eye movement desensitization and reprocessing therapy. I am hopeful that I can get to a point where the seizures stop altogether.

46

Person with PNES, USA

I am someone with many health conditions. The first was a moderate traumatic brain injury at five years of age. I was always told that I fractured my forehead during this fall. Over the years, I have had several other brain injuries, including one from playing football with friends and another from getting punched in the face. I also contracted viral meningitis at the age of twenty-one. I was hospitalized for two weeks for treatment. Then, at the age of thirty-two, I was again hospitalized with viral meningitis. They did a lumbar puncture and found herpes simplex virus in a polymerase chain reaction test and diagnosed me with recurrent viral meningitis, also known as Mollaret's meningitis. I continue to fight this disease to this day and believe it has become chronic instead of recurrent. I have a long list of traumas that I have experienced in my life. I had a bout with depression at the age of twenty-six that seemed to resolve. Then, at thirty-eight, I had a breakdown at work. I was on my first workbreak, and my wife could tell that I was losing it, and told me to come home. I lost it in my car and drove home sobbing uncontrollably (probably not a smart thing to do in hindsight). I got home and told my wife that I just couldn't do it anymore. Since then, I have tried to navigate the mental health system in the USA, and it has been a rough road. I haven't been able to find anyone to really help me. At age thirty-eight, I was also self-admitted to the mental health ward at the hospital for suicidal ideation. My family said that I was talking about suicide all the time and were worried about me, so I agreed to go. I was diagnosed with post-traumatic stress disorder, major depressive disorder, and generalized anxiety disorder. A couple of months after the hospitalization is when my non-epileptic seizures started, at age thirty-nine.

I had been separated from my wife and kids just prior to the hospitalization but had recently moved back in. We were trying to figure out where we were going to live because I had been terminated from my job since I couldn't go back to work, and social security disability and long-term disability had denied me, so we didn't have any income. One night, I was helping my wife pack, and it had been a long day. I was playing with my daughter and sat on the couch for a second to rest. My daughter asked me a question and I couldn't respond for some reason. Then I tried to open my eyes or move any body parts and I couldn't. I was trying as hard as I could to force my brain to make my body move, but it wouldn't. It really scared me. I had also had some seizure-type body movements a couple days earlier that I didn't think anything of until this event. I was under the care of a neurologist by now and called the on-call doctor. They said that it sounded like either seizures or sleep paralysis. They told me not to drive or climb ladders or anything like that until I could talk with my normal neurologist on Monday. I spoke with my neurologist on Monday, and an EEG test was ordered to determine if it was epilepsy. Luckily enough, my neurologist was an epilepsy specialist. The EEG test came back possibly abnormal to the left temporal lobe but not likely to be epilepsy. My seizures continued to get worse, though, with one event even lasting thirty minutes. Most are usually several minutes long. A seventy-two-hour ambulatory EEG test was ordered and showed no abnormalities at all, confirming that it wasn't epilepsy. That is when I received the official diagnosis of psychogenic non-epileptic seizures.

I have a wide variety of seizures, ranging from falling to the ground and having my extremities shake to episodes where everything goes blurry and my mind checks out for a little while. Most of my events lately are paralysis events. It starts with a sharp, shooting pain in my forehead or feeling really sleepy all of a sudden, generally meaning an event is going to happen. Most the time I can get to the ground before it happens, but sometimes I actually fall. During the events, I am aware of my surroundings and what is going on but cannot communicate. Every once in a while, I can grunt, but I can't talk, move, or communicate in any way. My wife is getting really scared that one of these times something more serious will occur and she won't be able to tell because she will believe that it is a non-epileptic seizure. She always checks to make sure that I am at least breathing. It is a really horrible situation. My kids even know what is going on because my four-year old daughter usually gets me a pillow and blanket to keep me comfortable and my one-year old son comes and gives me kisses.

One of the challenges I have with this diagnosis is that it seems like everyone wants to pass you off on to someone else. Neurologists send you to a psychologist because it is believed to be psychological. The psychologists, more often than not, don't know much about non-epileptic seizures, so they just try to treat any trauma and hope it helps. The challenge with the mental health industry is it is difficult to find qualified people to treat you. I had one that said I would be fine in several months. The next one was a neuropsychologist who said that I was in severe mental distress, but when I went to my psychologist, she said I was managing everything fine and didn't need any treatment. Then my most recent psychologist said she was wrong and that I did have problems, but she can't remember what we go over every week, so I have had to repeat myself several times. One of the challenges with the non-epileptic seizure diagnosis

PERSON WITH PNES, USA *(113)*

is attaching the psychogenic to it if it isn't epilepsy. I have Mollaret's meningitis, which some literature explains can be the cause of seizures. That was not considered, and I was given the psychogenic non-epileptic seizures diagnosis. I believe that if someone has an existing condition that says seizures are possible, then it would be considered before diagnosing psychogenic non-epileptic seizures. I have heard of people being diagnosed with psychogenic non-epileptic seizures, then finding out it is related to a heart condition, so it wasn't actually psychological. I believe that using the term *seizures*, until a definitive diagnosis can be made, would otherwise be a more appropriate terminology. I also believe that the naming system we have now is the way it is because the only test they have for seizures is to find out if it is epilepsy or not. So that has cornered us into using the term *epilepsy* or *non-epilepsy*. There are a lot of other conditions out there that have seizures as a related condition, so why not just start with seizures and, if you can narrow it down more, then change the diagnosis?

I was already unable to work before the seizures started happening, so it didn't cause me to lose a job or anything, but it has put a huge strain on family and friends. I don't have any friends that I go out and see. There are people that I communicate with online, but mostly in support groups for all of my conditions. My wife has to do pretty much everything because if I do too much, I end up having a seizure. That puts a huge strain on our marriage and her ability to stay calm with the kids. She has become the caregiver to a sick husband and two little kids. She doesn't get to go out and have fun with friends. She just writes because she is an author and trying to help support us and take care of us. She doesn't ever get personal time, and we rarely get couple time. That puts a huge strain on relationships. I have found that using a type of oil derived from the hemp plant has helped tremendously in controlling my seizures. That is another reason I believe that my seizures are more organic than psychological. I did a lot of research before trying this type of oil and had a couple of people I know who work in the psychology field recommend it, and it has been really helpful.

I hope that medical personnel learn to remember that most of us are not faking seizures and that they are freaking us out. We are not trying to cause them and are desperate for help. Be patient and kind toward us.

47

Mother Whose Daughter Has PNES, UK

My daughter has blacked out on and off since the age of thirteen—very intermittent initially, but since turning seventeen, this became increasingly worse. During the summer of 2015, it was a daily occurrence, often more than once a day. We saw many specialists and had many tests, including electroencephalography, electrocardiography, magnetic resonance imaging, and a tilt-table test. One private consultant we went to see thought that it was vasovagal syncope, but after a tilt-table test ruled this out. The latest diagnosis is that it is psychogenic nonepileptic seizures. We are not sure! It is happening less, but my daughter's general practitioner is still not comfortable to pass her as fit to work and therefore she is unable to work! When she blacks out, there is mainly no warning. She can be just walking along or sitting at a dressing table. When she goes, she can be out for up to five minutes. She is still, and when she comes back, she is often emotional and has a banging headache. During last summer, she broke her wrist, elbow, and ankle and dislocated her knee twice, resulting in surgery.

We are living this nightmare. We have sought a number of specialists and paid privately for one. She was receiving some benefit as she is unable to work, but this has now stopped as she was assessed as fit to work. Her general practitioner is fuming about this as she can absolutely not hold down a permanent role without letting anyone down!

She had a full-time job, which she had to give up. She was getting some incapacity support, which they have now stopped following an assessment.

48

Person with PNES, USA

For those of us who have survived the AIDS crisis since its inception, survival is plagued with overwhelming feelings of guilt and grief. The loss of most of my close friends was akin to being a shell-shocked veteran of war. I watched them fall one by one in rapid succession, and yet I stood helplessly by their bedsides as they withered and died. It was beyond what many, including myself, could endure.

My experience with AIDS began in the late 1970s, when I was in my early twenties. It was a time when it was difficult to maintain hope. We would have to wait almost two decades before we could see any significant slowing of this disease. Many could not bear the pain and found comfort in drugs, alcohol, or other methods to deal with the feelings of grief. I escaped in the form of a dissociative psychological disorder that for ten years was misdiagnosed as a form of epilepsy.

My misdiagnoses ranged from pseudotumor cerebri, myoclonus, idiopathic epileptic seizures, and finally, psychogenic non-epileptic seizures. My diagnosis was complicated and delayed by my fight with more life-threatening diseases, such as stage 3 large B-cell lymphoma and thyroid cancer. Those took priority, and my seizures just took a back seat. As long as I didn't have an episode during chemo, radiation, or a CT scan, they became more of an inconvenience to my doctors. I learned that the medical cannabis I took for chemo side effects also helped my seizures. The drugs that my doctors gave me were addictive and left me more like a zombie—a zombie doesn't complain. The main course of treatment prior to being diagnosed correctly was anti-anxiety and anti-epileptic drugs.

Once my fight with multiple cancers was won, I bounced from neurologist to neurologist trying different medications and modes of alternative medicine like acupuncture and biofeedback. Finally, I found a doctor that would administer a video-EEG test. This was the defining moment, when my doctor could see that my brain did not show any evidence of epileptic activity during a seizure.

It was difficult to receive the diagnosis. Being told that my seizures were all in my head made me feel as much of an outcast as my AIDS diagnosis. But I embarked on an intensive psychotherapy and psychiatric treatment. I was prescribed an anti-depressant to add to my complement of medical cannabis as a prophylaxis and an anti-anxiety drug for acute treatment during or at the onset of any episode.

It took about two years of treatment before I began to experience some changes. In the summer of 2016, my seizures took a strange turn. Up to this point, I would be able to find an escape during an episode by going someplace in my mind where I could not feel the pain from the contractions. But now I began to feel all the pain and stress during my episodes. I discovered that my back pain had a direct correlation to my episodes. Slowly, I learned how to breathe through an episode and prevent it from getting beyond what I was able to control.

Today, I am still in therapy. I wonder if I will ever reach the point of being seizure- and medication-free. It has been fifteen years since I went on disability. Looking back over the almost forty years of fighting to stay alive, it has been a long and difficult road, but somehow I think that I can finally see past today and am learning how to reclaim my life again.

49

Person with PNES, UK

I am a fifty-five-year-old, happily married lady with no children. I am the youngest of six children, with five older brothers. From a young age, I was sexually abused by my father until I was thirty-six years old, when he died. The psychological effect of that was dealt with over a period of five years using cognitive behavioral therapy techniques. At the end of this treatment, I was content that I had dealt with the abuse with no long-term effects remaining. This treatment ended toward the end of 2010. I had a close relationship with my mother, who passed away in September 2010. My nephew passed away in September 2012 due to a brain tumor. My second-eldest brother and father of my late nephew were killed in a road accident abroad in 2014.

My first seizure happened in October 2011. At first, I would occasionally experience a metallic taste before a seizure. The onset was very quick, not giving me time to lie down or take any safety precautions. I would often collapse to the floor, sometimes onto hard surfaces, causing serious injuries to my head and face. The initial seizures were long, with the longest being approximately ninety minutes. Due to the head injuries and the length of the seizures, I was admitted through Accident and Emergency to my local hospital. My initial admission lasted nearly ten weeks. During that time, I had several daily seizures of varying length. I understand that the ward medical team was so concerned on several occasions that they summoned the crash team [a team of doctors that responds to potential life-threatening emergencies]. I was treated with different anti-epileptic drugs as well as sedatives to calm the seizures. There was no discernable effect from the anti-epileptic drugs, but over the period, the seizures reduced in number and length, and so I was eventually discharged. I was readmitted for several more weeks soon after when the seizures stated again.

Throughout 2011 and 2012, I continued with seizures and sustained several serious facial injuries as a result of falling onto hard surfaces and/or banging my head repeatedly on the floor as part of the seizures. The metallic taste no longer pre-warned me. I had no indication of an onset, although my husband occasionally sensed a seizure coming on as he said that I went quiet and vacant. The seizures varied in length from seconds up to thirty minutes and most often occurred in a cluster of up to ten a time. After a seizure, when I came round, I felt vacant, disorientated, and confused. This would last about five minutes, and then I would need to go to bed to sleep for two or three hours due to extreme tiredness. I was frequently admitted through Accident and Emergency to the main hospital due to the injuries and seizures. Ambulance staff used the "scoop and run" approach and would administer a muscle relaxant intravenously to try and calm the seizures during the journeys to the hospital.

During my admissions, I was seen by several neurologists, and they continued with the epileptic approach until the middle of 2012, when a relatively newly qualified neurologist considered a further referral. She referred me to a professor as the only expert on the subject in the area. At the initial consultation with the professor, I was given a suspected diagnosis of non-epileptic attack disorder, but was referred for inpatient telemetry tests. The professor also asked my husband to video a seizure. Throughout this period, I had had tremendous support from my general practitioner, who also suggested videoing a seizure as he suspected something other than epilepsy. During my admission, a seizure was captured, and my husband had managed to video one previously. Consequently, the professor gave me a definitive diagnosis of non-epileptic attack disorder.

I can never explain how much of a relief it was to receive this diagnosis. Although I was told that there was no medical cure, I felt on cloud nine because I finally knew what was wrong with me. I had begun to get feelings that my local hospital doctors were becoming skeptical as I had not responded to any anti-epileptic drug. I was now in a position to say to them, "This is the illness I have, and this is how it should be treated." I was referred for a series of psychotherapy treatments, and I eventually had four sessions, but the therapist stated her main aim at that time was to get people to accept their diagnosis, which I had readily accepted. We did not continue with any further treatments at that time, although I have recently resumed them on the professor's advice.

Despite having a definitive diagnosis from the professor, I continue to have problems with this being accepted and understood at my local hospital. Although the professor had told me that non-epileptic seizures were not life-threatening, my husband still felt the need to call for assistance when I had prolonged seizures or injuries associated with them. Consequently, I continued to be admitted to wards, where I was given anti-epileptic drugs and sedatives until we produced a strongly worded letter from the professor indicating that this sort of approach would not help and could even be harmful. We had to be very forceful in our dealing with the doctors on this point.

I experienced some very disturbing attitudes and incidents over this period, which did not help with my condition:

1. A senior Accident and Emergency staff nurse remarking "that was good but I've seen better" to a junior doctor on seeing me having a seizure.

2. Medical admissions doctor: "Why have you had a seizure?"
   ME: "My brother has just been killed."
   DOCTOR: "Never mind, you're going home this afternoon."

3. Frequent references to "pseudoseizures," with the obvious inference that they are made up. Although I accept that this was the former term that was used, I felt intimidated by it. My husband researched the term and found that the World Health Organization had recommended that it be taken out of usage. I tried to educate medical staff about this, but with only limited success. Eventually, the Accident and Emergency doctors began to understand the nature of my illness and the information available. However, the ward doctors, especially the consultants, were less accepting. They seemed reluctant to research the available information or contact the professor or his team. My husband and I printed off and obtained all available information and passed it on to them. The professor had to provide several letters, the last one being strongly worded, to reinforce the diagnosis and treatment for non-epileptic attack disorder.

4. On one occasion, I attended Accident and Emergency with cuts to my arm and face. The triage staff nurse suggested that the cuts were due to self-harming.

5. Ambulance staff were among the most difficult to deal with. They seemed to latch onto the phrase "pseudoseizure," and many clearly used a layman's connotation of put-on or self-induced seizures. Only one or two of the senior technicians accepted our explanation of non-epileptic attack disorder and even took an interest in finding out more. The rest used the "scoop and run" method and insisted on administering sedatives until, finally, my husband pointed out that this could be harmful and they would be responsible.

6. As time wore on over the period of 2012 to 2015, relationships were built up with some of the Accident and Emergency doctors and staff so that admission to wards was restricted to head injuries rather than seizures. The hospital's dedicated epilepsy nurse took it on herself to further research and educate herself on non-epileptic attack disorder and then to educate healthcare professionals at the hospital. This had some effects, especially with younger staff, but older ones still seemed reluctant to progress.

7. After a strong disagreement with staff on a ward due to the treatment of myself and other patients, a meeting was arranged to put a care plan into place for any future admission. This plan covered treatment for associated injuries as well as correct monitoring of seizures and precautions to be taken.

   Since the action plan was formulated, I have managed to avoid admission. I have taken my own preventative measures, including moving to a new house. My husband has dealt with any facial injuries at home. The end of 2015 coincided with the conclusion of this process, which I believe also helped with the easing of my symptoms. I now suffer mainly with nighttime seizures, and the daytime ones are substantially reduced in length.

I have my own strongly held opinion about why my seizures started and their intensity. I use an analogy of a glass. My abuse filled the glass to the top with poison, but it did not overflow, and the treatment kept it below the top level. However, before my mother's passing, and with the passing of my nephew and brother in such terrible circumstances, the glass filled and overflowed. My own treatment at the hands of the medical staff and my battle with the hospital complaints system over five years continued to top up the glass so that it was constantly overflowing. It has only been since the satisfactory resolution of the complaints that the level in the glass is under some sort of control now. It has put a lid on the overflowing glass to a certain extent, although I continue with seizures still.

When I first started with seizures, any outgoing lifestyle was put on hold. I am a very gregarious person and never spent days in at home. After the seizures started, I rarely left my home, and both my husband and I were on constant watch for the onset of seizures. The only respite my husband had was when I was admitted to the hospital. Effectively, my life was on hold for twelve months. Following on from the professor's diagnosis, I had an overwhelming sense of relief. I knew what my illness was, how to treat it, and what to expect. I no longer doubted myself, and above all, I knew that it would not be life-threatening. I could explain my illness to family and friends, and brief them of what to expect and what action to take in the eventuality of me having a seizure in their presence. I was able to resume a sort of social life again, and I took every opportunity to go out. I had made a conscious decision that I would not let my lifestyle be dictated by my seizures, and that I would enjoy myself as much as I could despite the seizures. It is a cliché used by abuse sufferers, but I adopted the attitude that I was a survivor, not a victim. I took sensible precautions. I told everyone that I knew about the symptoms and treatment. I warned them to monitor me if I went quiet or looked vacant. I did not go out if I felt in any way that seizures were imminent. I never went out alone; at home, I stopped having baths and had a shower installed. My husband did the cooking so that I was not at risk from hot stoves or pans. I relished the chance to get on with my life again, albeit under close scrutiny.

Non-epileptic attack disorder as a diagnosis is still in its infancy. Newly qualified doctors seem to be accepting and knowledgeable about it, but the older doctors still have a problem with it. Even as recently as this year, one senior consultant persisted in calling my seizures "pseudo." Ambulance staff have not changed their attitude toward my seizures, and I am glad that I haven't had to call one this year. I am currently undergoing a further series of psychotherapy sessions. I feel that I am getting the most benefit from being open about the illness. I feel that I benefit from passing information to others, whether it is to health care professionals or the public about the illness. I want to help others with non-epileptic attack disorder and explain that it needn't be the end of your life, just something that can be managed in order to live a fuller life.

50

Partner of Person with PNES, UK

I am a sixty-two-year-old retired policeman and, as such, had some basic first aid knowledge. As part of my job, I dealt with some horrific sights and had to deal with some heartbreaking situations. However, nothing I ever did as a police offer was anywhere near as hard as having to watch my wife have seizures. The single most difficult experience was videoing a seizure in order to assist in her diagnosis.

When the seizures started, it was a massive shock. I had only ever witnessed one before in another person, and that one lasted a few minutes. My wife's first seizure lasted over an hour, and frankly, I was lost for what to do, except call for medical help.

On many occasions since, I have felt the same feeling of helplessness. Only since the diagnosis of non-epileptic attack disorder and learning that they are not life-threatening have I felt confident to deal with them on my own.

I had great faith in the medical system prior to the onset of the seizures, but as time wore on and nothing positive was found, I began to lose faith. The definitive diagnosis helped to restore some confidence, but as time has worn on and we have had the experiences we had with the medical system, I am lacking in confidence in it.

I do not know what it is like to experience a seizure, but it is pretty horrific to watch. The overall feeling is one of helplessness.

It may seem selfish, but I often think that it is somewhat harder to watch a seizure than undergo one, especially when they last for long periods.

Before the seizures started, I had witnessed firsthand the haphazard treatment of patients and noticed a marked difference in the approach to the treatment of elderly patients. In some instances, I would go so far to say that some staff (a very small minority) viewed the elderly as an inconvenience.

My wife saw this more than I did, firsthand as an inpatient, and was understandably upset.

I can see the link between the death of my mother-in-law, the onset of seizures, and the battle with the system. As the process failed to move forward, the seizures seemed to get worse, more prolonged, and violent. I tried to explain this potential link to the doctors and the complaints people, but no one listened.

On occasion, we were encouraged when the hospital "put procedures in place" or "took appropriate action to ensure things change," and it was pleasing to see that we had made a difference. But it was just as frustrating when we saw that these procedures were blatantly ignored or not actioned at all.

The diagnosis of non-epileptic attack disorder was truly an uplifting moment. It is not possible to describe the feelings we both had on our journey home from the consultant that day. At long last, we had received an answer, had a name for what the illness was, and we could now move forward both in our personal lives and re-garding our dealings with the system.

Before the diagnosis, I had been reluctant to leave my wife on her own. She had experienced seizures in the living room, in the garage (smoking area), and even while doing some gardening.

I had begun to be able to detect the beginnings of some seizures. The symptoms were her going very quiet, monosyllabic responses, or a vacant expression. On other occasions, she became overly talkative as if trying to distract herself from an onset.

The seizures themselves were characterized by twitching of her limbs and her head. It almost seemed like she was trying to bang the floor with her arms and head. She had some frothing to her mouth, and she was occasionally incontinent.

After coming out of a seizure, she would often almost straightaway go into an-other, again and again, with up to ten or more seizures after each other. At other times, one seizure would last an hour or more.

Finally, at the end of a seizure, or a cluster of seizures, she would appear vacant, disorientated, and unrecognizing of her surroundings or even me. This would last a few minutes, then she would feel tired and go to sleep, naturally, for a couple of hours.

The reluctance to leave her on her own and be overprotective lasted beyond getting the diagnosis of non-epileptic attack disorder. After the diagnosis, she made a conscious decision to get on with her life and not let the illness rule her. I had to admire her attitude, but I found it much more difficult to get on with things.

Even though the consultant had assured us that the seizures were not life-threatening and there was no treatment, I continued to use the emergency med-ical system, probably as a crutch. I just found it hard to sit by and watch her going through a seizure or seizures for long periods of time.

We finally agreed on a compromise; that is to say, if the seizures lasted over fif-teen minutes, then I should seek help. If there were any head injuries, then they took precedence. As time wore on, I extended the time that I was prepared to let the seizures last, and since December 2015, I have managed all seizures at home.

Much is said about the difficulty of being a carer, and I had not appreciated this before this illness. Our general practitioner provided fantastic support when we needed it, and my wife's positive attitude helped. But the sights of a seizure are such that it is very hard not to be on twenty-four-hour constant alert, and this is consequently debilitating for the carer. By twenty-four-hour constant alert, I mean going to bed after she had settled—often in the early hours, sleeping with one ear on the alert all the time, when sitting at home frequently glancing across to see if any of the telltale signs are evident. The results of these measures frustrated my wife. No matter how many times she told me to relax and deal with seizures if they happened, I could not relax, and it took the easing of the seizures to convince me, after five years.

Even now, I find myself glancing across when she is not looking, and I am a much later to bed and a lighter sleeper than I ever was.

Our experiences with the medical system were sometimes frustrating and often upsetting. It took considerable time, but we eventually established a good understanding with Accident and Emergency, especially as more newly qualified doctors came through the system and seemed more clued up on recently identified illnesses.

The neurology department at our hospital was trying, but not helpful, until the consultant's diagnosis, and then they seemed to be skeptical at first, followed by accepting and helpful once the epilepsy nurse had educated them more. I would stress that this is the appearance that they gave, and I may be wrong.

The admissions unit consultants were very hard to deal with, and even as recently as last December, they were still awkward. As an example, on one occasion my wife had been admitted to the ward with multiple long-lasting seizures. After five days, the seizures had subsided to one or two a day, but I could see that she was still lacking in confidence and generally feeling unwell. The consultant agreed that she would be kept until she went twenty-four hours without a significant seizure. The next day, a different consultant said that she would be discharged having gone twelve hours without a seizure. Despite my protests, he just stared arrogantly at me and said that they could do nothing for her on the ward.

Attitudes like this did nothing to give us confidence in the system, and I found it rocked my belief in the National Health Service. Specialists do not have this attitude, but the general admissions unit seems to suffer from this problem to a massive extent. As we talk to others on a regular basis, it seems that this is a generally held view—get people in and out as quickly as possible, with scant regards to the feelings of the patient.

Even with the letters that the consultant so kindly provided, the other consultants seemed reluctant to accept what was written. Although the consultant stated quite unequivocally that my wife's illness was real—that she was not putting it on, faking it, or harming herself with cuts—they continued to give an impression that they were the ones in charge and would make the decision. They were definitely unwilling to even ring him or his team for advice. At times, we had to be very forceful in putting our views across.

As a way of coping with all we have been through over the last five years, we have decided that helping to improve things for others is the way to move forward.

We have helped to produce a video for the training of staff dealing with patients and their care, and about compassion and communication—topics we feel that hospitals have let us down on most.

We have been delighted to help with studies aimed at furthering investigations of non-epileptic attack disorder and with obtaining further funding for these investigations. We have been further delighted to be part of the first case study into non-epileptic attack disorder for the *British Medical Journal*. Contributing to this book has been helpful, and we will be delighted to help or meet others who might be involved in dealing with this illness.

The best advice I could hope to give to anyone in our position is to deal with it as a couple, don't let the illness rule your life, take what help there is from the experts who know what they are on about, and finally, do not let the system grind you down.

As investigations continue into the illness, the knowledge will pass down the system, but it seems that widespread knowledge will take some time to get "out there" unless a celebrity is diagnosed and publicizes the illness or someone takes up the cause.

51

Person with PNES, UK

I have been living with non-epileptic seizures since June 2013, and I was officially diagnosed in August 2013. My current diagnosis is functional neurological disorder with non-epileptic seizures. This has affected every aspect of my life. I am no longer able to teach full-time and barely manage to teach part-time. I have two children, both boys, aged ten and fourteen. Unfortunately, having witnessed my deterioration firsthand, both my boys have experienced some mental health issues. I am lucky to have a really supportive partner. However, I know that my illness has had an impact on him also.

It has been a long, hard road, and I am yet to see a major improvement when trying to live a relatively normal life. I believe that in order to try and manage non-epileptic seizures, you have to try and learn to "read" the signs that your body is under too much pressure. My warning signs include: a continuous debilitating migraine, a strange tingling and burning sensation all over my body, and a general tremor. Sometimes, the warnings give you time to get to a safe position, but other times the warnings are very brief.

Another thing that is really important when living with non-epileptic seizures is to not overwork (this is extremely difficult in my profession). If I become exhausted, my seizures increase heavily. In an ideal world, I would take a long period off from work, but my financial situation doesn't allow for that. I am very fortunate to still be able to work living with functional neurological disorder and non-epileptic seizures as I know that many others are unable to. However, the result of still working means that my family suffers because I am generally very ill most evenings.

One way I have learned to cope with and accept my non-epileptic seizures is by writing a blog to help spread awareness. Through the blog, I have found many other sufferers and have had the chance to share my story with others who can support me. I hope all this information helps. In reality, non-epileptic seizures are an awful thing to live with as there is currently no cure and the neurological physiotherapy only holds the seizures off until later in the day. I think that it's important to always try and find the positives in your situation, and that, along with my fantastic partner and lovely children, are what gets me through each and every day.

52

Person with Epilepsy and PNES, UK

My seizures started a year ago; they have had an impact on every area of my life. Mostly work: I tried to continue to work and have fought hard to stay, but I have faced bullying and discrimination, which in turn increased the seizures. Before a seizure, I get a headache, then I start to twitch, my mouth first, then my body jerks. I can't respond to anyone around me. Sometimes I lose bladder control. Other times they are short, and I come out with a jumbled brain unable to recall words or focus. I'm often dizzy for some time after, and I need to sleep. Moneywise, it is difficult. I often have to pull out of social occasions.

53

Person with Epilepsy and PNES, UK

I went to my expert neuropsychiatrist, and he said something like "I am diagnosing you with a dissociative disorder. You are distant from the world. Although you have epilepsy, what you are experiencing are not epileptic seizures. You are having pseudo-epileptic seizures. You are depressed. You have had some trauma in your life that needs to be unearthed. Take some anti-depressants, exercise, eat well, plan to do something exciting, and come back in three months' time when you have figured out what's wrong with you. I will put you on a waiting list to see a therapist in six to nine months' time."

I know he's a supersmart doctor, but I'm not convinced by what he said. So I am still on my search down the crumbling dirty track road, looking for my pot of gold. However, diagnosis is key, and I believe his diagnosis—that I am dissociative—is correct, though I am not convinced of the cause. But I have now been given the name of an expert in dissociative disorders, and I am trying to track him down.

I have epilepsy as well, and I wouldn't know how to differentiate between an epileptic or non-epileptic seizure.

54

Person with Epilepsy and PNES, UK

I have been experiencing seizures for the last eighteen months. I was first diagnosed in April 2015. At first, I was confused about why this was happening to me, then it was explained that I could be having these seizures due to a past traumatic experience. My past experience is being sexually abused by my half-brother. I was confused about why it was happening now, and it was explained to me that sometimes it starts when your mind is at rest.

When I started having these seizures, my mind was at rest. This is because two months earlier, he was sent to prison, and I had moved away. I felt safe. Having these seizures has changed my life completely, and my plans for my life have changed. I was working as a support worker before I moved away, but now I am unable to work as my seizures are uncontrolled. I feel scared to walk out of the house on my own as I am scared that I am going to hurt myself and end up in Accident and Emergency. I thought that as my half-brother was in prison, I could get on with my life and not have to worry about walking out my front door. I was far from right. I didn't know anyone who had this condition, and I didn't know what this condition was. I was given the name of a website by my neurologist where I could read up about this condition.

I have been told by a number of health care professionals that these seizures are all in my head and that I am making them up. That is a lie. I would do anything to go back to work. I started off by having seizures where I stare into space and was having up to thirty each day. Then I was having seizures where I would drop to the floor. Now I have seizures that mimic tonic-clonic seizures. In between these, I lose my speech. I also have functional dystonia in my left foot. This makes it very difficult to walk and move around. I now have about three seizures a day. I never used to get a warning for them, but I am starting to now. My warnings are where my stomach feels like it is being turned upside down and I get a fog over my eyes. The next thing I remember after that is coming round and feeling really achy. I have had the paramedics out a few times, and some of them have been helpful but others have not. I just want to try and control my seizures and get on with my life.

To anyone out there with these seizures, I just would like you to know that you are not alone. There are more people out there with these seizures than you think. You are not alone.

55

Person with Epilepsy and PNES, USA

I was diagnosed with epilepsy at eighteen months old. My parents were divorced by age five, and both remarried. Later into my mother's second marriage, she left, and she started a relationship with another woman. We moved in with this other woman. It is then that my severe physical and mental abuse started. My mother just watched and stood by as her partner abused only me, and not my siblings because they were still toddlers. This went on for many years.

I eventually ended up in foster care, while my siblings were left in the home. I was in foster care for a few years before my mother came and said if I don't return, I'll never see her again. As a pre-teen, that's a thought that I didn't want. So I returned home. Unfortunately, the abuse restarted again, this time for two years. I was then placed in the foster care system again. My first night there, I was sexually assaulted by someone at night. As a "new kid," I felt I had no standing at the children's home where I was. I never told anyone of that first night there. I was then admitted into a foster family home, where I lived until I was of age that I had to leave. At that time, I was reintroduced back to my mother and family. I told my mother that the only way I would come home is if her new partner would never abuse me again.

At this time, I was seventeen years old. I graduated from high school and attended a vocational school for the disabled. There I studied business management and received something similar to an associate's degree. Even searching for a job afterward, no one wanted to hire me because of my seizure disorder.

Ten years went by, and I had an occipital lobectomy for my seizure disorder. I was warned against the procedure because it could take more of my vision away. I was already legally blind, but that didn't matter to me. I was having more than two hundred seizures a week. After the procedure, the doctors and myself were shocked that my vision improved to 20/30 vision! I could get rid of my white cane. I had met my future wife just two years prior through a blind bowlers league. We married two years after my surgery. She has been my rock ever since. I seriously do not know where I would be without her by my side. This year, we will be married twenty-five years.

I was diagnosed with psychogenic non-epileptic seizures in 2005; the doctors there who made the diagnosis did not treat me very well. It was then that both my wife and I were looking for answers to pseudoseizures as they called them. I was told that I never was or will be an epileptic, and that I faked all my seizures for attention. I then told the specialist that I guess they give anyone brain surgery and a vagal nerve stimulator just because. It has been a very long eleven years after the diagnosis. It has taken me longer to accept than I thought. We are very active raising awareness to all. I still have seizures. I'm told it's because I can't forgive my mother for what she allowed to happen. She is deceased now, and I can't confront her personally.

56

Mother Whose Daughter Has PNES, UK

I am the mother of a fifteen-year-old girl, who was diagnosed with non-epileptic attack disorder in October 2016. It has been a very long journey. Through this horrid journey, my daughter has had two so-called specialist neurologists. She was diagnosed with epilepsy, jerking limbs, and restless leg, to name a few. She has had three MRI scans and twice had a two-hour EEG test (which I do not think was long enough). I was told by one neurologist that there is nothing that she can do for my daughter as it's not medical but I can still see her if you wish!! When we were seen by the Child and Adolescent Mental Health Services, we were told that she has no mental health issues. This has been an uphill battle, and if my daughter did not have mental health issues before, with this condition and the way that the medical professionals have treated myself and my daughter, believe me, she will—given the fact that they are not aware of the condition, and their attitude that she must be putting it on or she is an attention seeker.

When I recently had an appointment with both of her neurologists, I was told that I don't have to waste the time of the hospital staff and my time taking her up to the hospital, even if she has had a very long and violent seizure (also a word I CANNOT use . . . look up the description in the English dictionary, I bloody well will). Basically, if I feel that I need to take her up there, I will.

57

Person with Epilepsy and PNES, USA

I began having seizures after a car accident that left me in a coma for a month. I have both epileptic and non-epileptic seizures. Also, I have post-traumatic stress disorder. I get these awful auras that lead to grand mal seizures. In the summer, it's worse. I feel that stress has something to do with these. I moved to a new city for a year a few years back, and I did not have one aura or even a panic attack while living there. I rented a room and had more concerns to worry about. But I never felt depressed. As soon as I moved back home with my parents, they began. I feel depressed. I get awful auras and tremors that won't let me sleep. I was taking medication that would not help much versus their endless side effects. I now smoke cannabis to keep these under control. I can't get rid of them completely, but wonder why when I moved to a new city I went more than a year without one. I also have applied for disability and been denied three times.

I need help.

58

Person with PNES, UK

Tomorrow morning, I am driving for an appointment with my consultant. My old consultant has moved on, so I'm unsure who will be seeing me, and I need to make sure that I spend some time thinking and processing what I want to ask them, and what exactly they can do to help me get back to some form of normality as the previous techniques haven't been working so well.

No one will be with me at the appointment, which is fine, but sometimes I don't always hear correctly what they are saying, or understand and remember everything properly after they've gone. My mum was going to come, but she's supervising my sister, who is still waiting for an operation on her shoulder. I haven't seen a consultant since last year, and I have had very little input from the center since my recent flare-up.

I guess the difficulty with these meetings is that the time and resources the hospitals have compared to what you think you need don't always match up. I also have to travel nearly two hours for my appointment as this is the nearest center for treatment for my condition. Sadly, this isn't particularly pleasant; however, it's always worth it when you know you have someone who understands a little more about what you're going through. I have an amazing physiotherapist who I've been able to see privately. I love how she has more time out of the National Health Service and totally understands functional neurological disorders way more than most other physiotherapists, and can work with the bizarreries of my own body; this is especially true when we consider how often a patient with functional neurological disorder can override their difficulties walking and do something like running or cycling with no problems at all. I've been amazed and astounded how weird, but encouraging, it is to still be able to do some of these things. The problems tend to lie in what society perceives when I'm thinking about going running from home. I worry about my neighbors seeing me in a wheelchair to go up into town, and the questions posed seem to stop me from wanting to have a go at running, which is annoying for me. That said, in some ways, it's none of their business, and I've always been really lucky that my awesome physiotherapist has been encouraging me all the time to do some of my old activities despite my walking problems. It's very tricky to plan activities nowadays as twenty-four hours can be very different depending on how you are feeling in the morning, or at various points of the days. Friends have got used to me canceling things last minute, or indeed not being able to meet up, simply because the overstimulation or conversation or activities exhaust me in mind and body. I know that I need "time out" and spend time on the sofa to try and recover when I get to that stage. For example, I started to experience some bad pain in my arms at the holiday club this morning, which was a bit of a sure sign that things weren't going so well. When that happens, I have to act quickly to get in rest and recuperation, and this often means alone time. If not, I can end up worse off. However, this then makes me feel like I've become extremely anti-social and very boring to be around. When I do try and ignore symptoms, it often comes back to bite me, and I know I need to keep trying, but sometimes it's really hard to motivate knowing the consequences of doing an activity. It's that funny thing about your mind/body relationship, though, because your mind knows, and then gets into a pattern and response of *I've done something hard, therefore I need to rest.* However, I'm not sure if this is always the case. The sofa I am lying down on was bought to help me rest, and there is a particular dent in just one place where I always lie down to put my feet up. This makes me laugh as I always sit in one place so that I can see the television and the gorgeous view of the country park outside, which sometimes has cattle on my eye level as I'm on the top of three floors of the house.

I know I need to write some things down to take to the consultant tomorrow. As I am hopeless in that, I always try and put on a brave face and say that everything is fine, when actually things really aren't. I hate wasting their time, and I hate being a bother, and I never want to be one of those really annoying, complaining people that they have to deal with. Having doctors galore in my family has probably influenced this (mum, dad, and big sister at the moment; oh, and an aunty!). I guess also it comes down to that some people are much worse off, but there is a lot of negativity and complaining and *I'm so bad, let me tell everything about me* on the internet. I started a blog up for this time round in my symptoms, partly as I thought it would help my friends understand a little more of the intricacies of what's going on, but also so that there was something more positive in how to deal with functional neurological disorders rather than, *Wow, this is so dreadful, isn't it?*

59

Person with PNES, USA

I'm a thirty-year-old mother to a very bossy and beautiful daughter. I am surrounded by the most amazing family and friends anyone can ask for. On April 3, 2015, I woke up paralyzed from the waist down. Then began my LONG, LONG journey to figuring out what was going on. After over thirty hospital stays for EEG tests, twelve MRI scans, ten CT scans, two lumbar punctures, two surgeries, electroshock therapy, and many other tests, we received a diagnosis of a rare condition: conversion disorder.

I have dealt with almost every aspect of this condition. Paralysis, loss of speech, loss of memory, fainting, not being able to eat, and what I consider to be the worst: the uncontrollable seizures. You know it's pretty bad when the ambulance shows up and almost every paramedic knows you on a personal level now. I cannot explain the embarrassment and shame. As of 2015, I could no longer work due to multiple seizures and 911 [the emergency number for the US] calls from my job. I have taken every medication under the sun to try and treat this condition. Unfortunately, insurance will not cover most of the VERY HELPFUL treatments for this condition. Doctors have loaded me up with anti-anxiety pills, anti-depressants, sedatives, and every calming medication out there to simply make me a shell of the funny, outgoing person that I used to be. But as we all know, alternative medicine is not something the insurance companies want to pay for. I have slowly began treatments but cannot afford them any longer. Between rent, groceries, and just life itself, some treatments have taken the back seat. My family has given almost all. These medical treatments have left me like a zombie or medical guinea pig, and I want to actually try to overcome this and be myself again!

60

Person with PNES, USA

Last year, I was an activity director at a nursing home. My job was physically, emotionally, and mentally draining and was an hour and a half away from my home, but I loved it. I had so much passion for what I did, and the work brought me great joy. The commute and stress had been building for months, so I had considered a new job, but my employer came up with a great strategy to reduce my hours and I stayed on. I began having a significant intention hand tremor when doing fine motor tasks, such as putting in my earrings or eating without a table for support. I had always had some tremor. It ran in my father's side of the family. This tremor was much more prominent, and when I started to have a neck tremor, I became concerned. The neck tremor came on when I was speaking or eating. As the month went on, it was getting worse and worse. I went to see my physician's assistant, and she referred me to a neurologist. The neurologist diagnosed me with essential tremor. She told me to stay away from caffeine and gave me a prescription for a beta-blocker. That is where my harrowing story begins.

The day after I took the medication, on recommendation from my doctor I returned to work. I had a tremor in the morning but felt well enough to lead my exercise class with the twenty or so residents. I would instruct everyone on the various exercises and model it for them, and then we would repeat, and then I would assist those that couldn't do the exercises on their own. Midway through the class, I tried to tell everyone the next exercise, but my neck began to tremor, and this time I could not speak. I tried again to no avail. I rested a few moments and yet again could not speak. The residents were getting anxious, and I was unable to offer much comfort. There were moments that I could speak and times that I could not, but it seemed that finishing the class was out of the question. I waved my coworker over, and she helped get another program started while I rested in the office. My peers were informed, and they suggested I go home. I decided to stay and just do office work as the commute was so long and I wasn't really sure what was going on with my body. Besides, essential tremor was something that I was going to have to learn to deal with. It would not go away. I tried leading a bingo game that afternoon, and like before, I had done well for a while, but a bingo ball dropped on the ground. I bent to pick it up, and then my neck began to tremor and I was mute. I decided to leave early and discussed my issue with our Director of Nurses, and he said that the beta-blocker would take a few days to start working. Being Christmas week, the busiest week of the year for a Christian-based nursing facility, I decided to try to work again the following day. I did not make it very far this time.

What I didn't know is that it would be my last day of work. I was able to finish the exercise class, but afterward, I felt funny. It was like I had tunnel vision. I started to walk toward the nurse's station, and afraid that I would fall down, I just held onto the counter. A housekeeper noticed me standing there not looking well, so she pulled up a chair and rolled me behind the nurse's station and went to go get help. My hand was tremoring a little, but I felt like something was very wrong. The Director of Nurses came up and started yelling at me to go home, that I shouldn't be at work. She pulled me into my office and started directing people to cover for me with the residents and to call my husband. My boss came in to talk to me, and my neck would tremor and I couldn't speak at times, and then my arm started repeatedly moving. It was circling around and slapping my leg repetitively. It would happen like the tremor, in waves and then stop, start and then stop. We both decided that this was likely seizure activity. I was not new to seizures as my son had been diagnosed with epilepsy two years prior. However, my symptoms were nothing like his. The seizure activity continued until they found me a place to lie down alone in the dark, and they dissipated.

My husband arrived and then drove me toward the hospital. I still felt "off." Something was just not quite right, and then my torso dropped and my arms and neck started to thrash. Further evidence that now I too might have epilepsy. I had a few more spells before we got to the hospital and then another when the paramedics came out to get me from the bench outside the hospital. They got me into a room, and different doctors and nurses and staff were coming in and out and asking questions and taking blood and putting in the intravenous line and hooking electrodes up to my chest. I continued to have these spells. The doctor came in and had me touch my nose and then touch his finger. When I would try to reach out, I would start to seize. They had me go to x-ray and get a CT scan. Then they gave me an anti-epileptic drug and a muscle relaxant. Things settled, and they sent me home with a prescription for an anti-epileptic drug and an appointment with their neurologist.

Christmas morning, I awoke seizing. This time, it was my whole body. My husband called the hospital, and they had me go back to the Emergency Room. The CT scan had shown a cyst at the back of my skull that they wanted to check, so they gave me more muscle relaxant and sent me in for an MRI, which showed a lesion in my left frontal lobe. The seizures continued, so they started trying various seizure medications on me. One type caused tremendous pain as it entered my arm and moved up my shoulder. I had them stop it. They tried a slower drip, but I was still feeling pain. They then tried a different type, which went in better but caused tinnitus, where it sounded like every sound was robotic, and I felt like my insides were itchy but there was no outer rash. I had always been sensitive to medications, but this was the first time that I had an allergic reaction. They finally prescribed two types of seizure medication with a muscle relaxant and an anxiolytic.

My symptoms took a turn for the worse. I started having aphasia, which was a speech issue that I was accustomed to from my residents at the nursing home but something I had never experienced myself. I also had more times when I couldn't speak, what I now know as apraxia. I couldn't even say my name. The seizures increased as well. I could almost count on them several times a day. I would have out-of-control intention tremor when I tried to eat or use my hand or fingers for any fine motor tasks. I became very sensitive to lights and sound, especially the fluorescent lights in the hospital. They all brought on seizures, even the television. The tables had turned, and I had become the patient. The staff ran several EEG tests, but my movements caused them problems and they were unable to record any anomalies. The neurosurgeon decided to do a biopsy of the lesion. I had the surgery, and on top of all my seizure and anxiety medications, they put me on a pain medication, and at some point, they added an anti-depressant to the mix. I slept all the time, and when I wasn't sleeping, I was on edge due to the speech and motor issues and of course the seizures.

A few days after the surgery, when they had found nothing distinct about the lesion except that it was fourteen millimeters of abnormal cells, they decided to transfer me to another hospital to have a video-EEG test. As I was leaving the hospital, they did not give me my routine medications, and I traveled to a neighboring city in the back of an ambulance. When I arrived, they brought me in, and again, a myriad of doctors and nurses came in asking questions, running tests, and started to hook electrodes up to my head with smelly glue. I had asked them to keep the lights off above my head, but they needed them for the electrodes, so after a short time in the fluorescent lights with all the other sensory overstimulation, I began to seize. My family asked them to bring my medications, but the doctors said that there was no medication order yet, so I kept seizing. My husband had gotten kicked out of the room for yelling at the nurses as they tried to do their job. We were all stressed. My husband came back in and held my hand, reminding me to breathe. I usually forgot to breathe when the seizures came on, so I frequently needed that reminder. He told me to think about a trip we had taken to the beach with our son. He told me to remember our son playing in the rocks and waves, looking for jellyfish and crabs. That helped calm me, and the seizure slowed. That image of my son in that still moment in time got me through many seizures.

Why weren't the doctors and nurses helping me? It felt like forever, hours even. I found out later that the seizure was only twenty minutes in duration. Those twenty minutes sure did feel like forever. A night filled with panic attacks, headache, anxiety, nausea, mind racing, and what I now know as brain zings and part of what is called withdrawal syndrome followed. The nurse finally gave me part of my prescriptions, and then the doctor came in and diagnosed me with anxiety. They said that I was to go home on an anxiolytic. But what about the speech and neuromotor issues, what about the lesion, what about the seizures? It was no longer a neurological problem; it was a psychological problem and therefore not their problem. I was discharged. My mom and my aunt had come out to help take care of me, so I was not alone. But they did need to get back to their lives. My mom is a nurse and my aunt a postal worker, so they were counted on for their jobs and for their families.

I went to see my neurologist for a follow-up, and she came in an hour late and said, "You just have anxiety. Continue to take the prescription, and go see a psychiatrist and find a therapist." She gave me a list of referrals and told me to make an appointment for a check-up in six months. "But what about the aphasia? What about the neuromotor issues, what about the seizures?" I asked. She said to discuss it with the psychiatrist. So I did. The psychiatrist had no idea what to do with me. I shared my story, and she had the most confused look on her face. She asked many questions, and I spoke when I could, and my husband filled in where I couldn't. She referred me to a neuropsychologist and recommended that I try to wean off of the anti-anxiety medication. To make the process easier, she prescribed an anti-depressant to be taken daily. I had a seizure in the car after the appointment. I went to the therapist as also prescribed. She gave the same confused looks, discussed my possible anxiety triggers (which were the symptoms), and told me to start writing everything down in a journal. She said to me that there was definitely something else wrong and also referred me to a neuropsychologist. I am grateful to both for their advice. The addition of a different drug was another story. I tried tapering off of the anxiolytic, but each time I did, I ended up with worse seizures, worse neuromotor function, and worse speech. My psychiatrist recommended that I stay on the medications until I could see a neurologist. In the meantime, the neuropsychologist did two days of cognitive testing with me. She found issues that I didn't even know I had. I couldn't write a slow line across a piece of paper. I was very slow with the motor cognitive tests even when I thought I did great. I had spells and seizures in her office as we did the testing but made it through. She also did psychological testing on me, trying to determine if the underlying cause was anxiety. She did not think so from my results and forwarded the results to my neurologist. My neurologist was not supportive of her work, or of my health, so I found a new one.

Meanwhile, my mom and aunt had returned to their home state, and I was left to my own devices. I couldn't drive, but I had great neighbors that helped me get around. I had some difficult moments, but with each one, I learned more about my condition and more about my triggers. I learned to keep my medications nearby in an easy-to-open case and to set an alarm to remind me to take them. I learned that I could go to public places only if I wore earbuds to block the excess noise and sunglasses under the fluorescent lights and that I could never be left in public alone. I learned that I needed to pace my day so as to not fatigue my brain. When I was tired, my symptoms were worse. One seizure would exhaust me for hours.

I had to rest after each one in a dark and quiet place. My husband ended up getting me fancy headphones that block outside noise. I used them regularly. I received physical therapy, occupational therapy, and speech therapy. They taught me ways of coping. I had to slow down and use rhythm for my speech and for motor tasks. They taught me deep breathing and other anti-anxiety techniques, such as guided meditation, guided relaxation, and yoga. I also needed to learn to recognize when a task was becoming too much before it brought on a seizure.

My physical therapist found some new issues: clonus, a resting tremor in my legs, and spasticity, a curling in of my right foot when trying to look back and forth while walking. I saw my new neurologist, and she was just as confused by my issues as everyone else. She prescribed me a small dose of an anti-epileptic daily because of my brain lesion and the likelihood that I might actually have epileptic seizures. She did not want me to go off of either of the other medications. I tried this drug a couple of times, but it just increased my hypersomnia. As it was, I would sleep most of the day. My mom had been asking for me to go up north to one of the university hospitals. I couldn't get an appointment at the university hospital near me, so I decided to go. I wasn't getting anywhere here. My loving husband took three days to drive me there and three days to drive back alone. I made an appointment with the most prestigious school that I knew. I tried to schedule an appointment with the neuromotor specialist, but they kept referring me to the epileptologist, which I thought was strange because they had already ruled out epilepsy. When I got to my mom's house, the spasticity had gotten worse. It started to affect my regular walking. It got so bad that my mom had to borrow a walker from the nursing home where she worked. I went to the Emergency Room, and they had a multitude of doctors come see me. They did the same neurological exams that I always failed and that brought on seizures, such as the point to your nose and point to my finger test. They eventually determined that I was safe to go home. So again I was discharged, using the borrowed walker.

I had been suffering from allergies for the past month, and I had been taking some different allergy medicines. I started to realize that this was making me sleep far too long, so I switched to another, which my pharmacist had approved as safe with the medications that I was on. I didn't notice it then, but the medications that I was taking were progressively making me worse. I started having severe seizures often, and with the fact that I could barely walk, it was starting to get dangerous for me to be alone. We contacted the epileptologist, and we were able to get me admitted into the hospital for another video-EEG test. This time, it went a lot smoother. It was not as chaotic, and they did not make any changes to my medication schedule, at least at first. After two days on the EEG test, they determined that my seizures were non-epileptic, and they moved me to the psychiatric unit at the hospital. There was a team of doctors and medical students working with me daily. The fellow neurologist insisted that my symptoms were caused by anxiety, and he stated that there must be something that triggered it. I could think of no possible triggers, so we were both frustrated. I told him that it might be useful to see what I was like off of the medications. So we found out. Unbeknownst to me, he took me off the anti-anxiety medication. I started to have an increase in episodes, but I was no longer on video, so I was to press the button when I had a seizure and wait until a staff member came. The staff was much less responsive to my call bell. I was not supposed to get up by myself to use the restroom, but had I waited I would have had an accident each time. There were now more important patients. My arm folded up on itself one morning. I reported it to the nursing staff, but it is not documented anywhere on my records. Nor is the entire day that I spent with facial seizures and increased full body seizures that eventually led up to dystonia, where my body started curling up tightly over to my right side, starting with my neck. It was very painful and would turn into a full-body seizure. When I had company, they would press the button and the nurse would come in, but when I was by myself, I had to figure out how to lift my head back up on my own. The muscles in my neck would not help me to reposition, so I had to pull my head up with my hands. My tongue started to fold up inside my mouth, and I would start to seize and I couldn't breathe. The nurse came in during one of the episodes and had to roughly turn my body over. I felt like I might swallow my tongue. When I would speak, eat, drink, or move, it triggered the dystonia, which triggered the seizures. Thankfully, my parents came that night and called the doctor to have them do something. There was an on-call doctor that had come in. The doctor addressed my parents and immediately started talking to them about me like I wasn't in the room. They conversed while my neck and body were contorting, and it was like I wasn't there. At one point, I asked if someone could lift up my head. At another, I raised my voice and said, "What about me? What about the patient? I have some questions!" That brought on another seizure as she continued to talk to my parents and then asked them to join her in the hallway where I could hear them discuss my anxiety and the psychological history of my family, including a brother who had a nervous breakdown at eighteen and a grandmother who had schizophrenia. She got me a dose of an anxiolytic, and my symptoms began to settle. I still couldn't eat or drink, and I was very dehydrated. I had a splitting headache, nausea, and brain zings, which I can only describe as my brain was scrambled. My thoughts moved so fast to irrelevant things that made no sense. It was like I was going crazy. The nurse refused to give me a painkiller for the headache, since it was not on the doctor's order. The facial seizures continued, and at times it was like I was baring my teeth like an animal. Other times my tongue would protrude, and I would start to seize. At one of these moments, an aide came in and put the thermometer into my mouth. As I was seizing, she was writing down my stats on the board and entering information on the computer. She took the oxygen sensor off of my finger and removed the thermometer without once looking at me. She had no idea I was seizing. She never stopped to look. Early the next morning after a night of no sleep, I had pressed my call bell because I had to use the bathroom. I pressed it again when no one came. And yet again. I did not dare move, as I was still having seizures with the merest movement and still couldn't eat or drink. The nurse came in, and I told her that I needed assistance. She sent her aide in, and she went to get me out of bed. I said that I couldn't. She responded, "Oh, now you're going to use the bedpan, huh!" She ripped the covers off and placed the bedpan in an agitated manner. When I finished and hadn't moved, she roughly wiped me and stormed out, like I was a criminal, like I wanted her to help me go to the bathroom on purpose. I felt dirty. I felt hurt. I felt neglected and alone. No one understood.

I finally dozed a bit, and like many times since December, I was praying. Praying for help and praying for answers. As the day set in, I started to feel clarity of mind. My mind had not been that clear since everything began. It was now May, and for the first time, I felt normal. The seizures stopped. My speech was improving. I could get up, get dressed, and walk. I heard the team of medical staff outside my door discussing me and how they were going to present me my diagnosis. They talked about how I didn't appear to have suicidal thoughts, so it should go smoothly. With a clear head, I was ready. They came in and crowded around me like they had every morning, and before they could speak, I said, "You know, I think this could have been caused by anxiety from overworking myself between my commute, job, and family life. I suspect the medications have made it worse." The fellow doctor responded, "You are going home off of the anxiolytic, so you should feel much better." His superior, the attending, reprimanded him for taking me off of the medication so fast. "You can't do that!" he said. "That can cause a lot of problems." I heard him continue discussing it with him after they left the room. It clearly did cause a lot of problems as I continued to have withdrawal symptoms for the next week. Fortunately, they were not as bad as the night with the dystonia. That will forever remain as the worst night of my life. The attending told me that they were going to have to discharge me that day. I couldn't stay anymore, and rehab facilities would not take me, so I had to go home. "What about the seizures? What about the dystonia?" It didn't matter. I had to go home in whatever state I was in because this was a psychological issue and not a medical issue. With a clear head, I called my family and let them know so that they could set up the arrangements. They were worried, but we all had no choice. They put me back on the anxiolytic daily so that hopefully the withdrawals would not bring on the dystonia again. The fellow doctor came into my room in the evening by himself. He said that it was not possible that my seizures had come from overworking myself. He said it had to be a trauma. I must be suppressing something. Then he left. It was like he had to get that off his chest before he went home for the day. A psychiatrist came in and said that I should look into my anger issues. The only time I had been angry was when I yelled at the doctor for ignoring me. I think there were other issues that needed to be looked at. I met with the head of the department the following morning. He was wonderful, and even though I was late for my appointment and he had already left the building, he returned to speak with me and spent over an hour listening to me, explaining my condition, and giving me advice. He was one of the first medical doctors in the whole experience that actually listened to me. He told me that it was possible that there was no direct trauma and that I had been misinformed. There was no reason that I couldn't have caused myself great anxiety by my lifestyle.

I went home and improved, slowly trying things I couldn't do before and finding that I could do them. A series of successes! I felt better, clearer, and happier than I had been. I started going on day trips with my family, to restaurants, and to stores. I wasn't completely fixed. I still needed to get off of the medication. But I was better and I returned home to my husband and son. When I tried to taper off of the medication, under another psychiatrist's guidance, I had my first seizures in over a month. The psychiatrist kept saying that she didn't understand why I was having such bad responses to withdrawal. If she didn't understand, then who did? Her lack of knowledge was causing me great discomfort during my withdrawals, as the tapers were too much for my body to handle. My neuropsychologist helped me to taper more so than my psychiatrist, by microtapering. She told me to just scrape a bit off of the pills every day, which worked much better. I still needed someone that could understand the withdrawal aspect of the drugs. I went to see my primary care physician to update him on everything and to see if he could help me. He decided to do a DNA test on me to see if my problem wasn't just part of my genetic code. The results came back and, as it turns out, I am a rapid and ultrarapid metabolizer of certain medications. Because of this, my body stores up toxins from these medications. The medications I had been taking were all on that list. I had been poisoned by the drugs that were supposed to help me. It is part of a new science called pharmacogenetics. For this science, I am grateful, as otherwise I would have never known. I am slowly regaining my independence. I am still tapering off of the medications, as I am among the one in four that suffer from withdrawal syndrome from some of the medication and I have bad side effects each time I cut down. Who knows what issues I will have when I have eliminated the medications completely. Will I have seizures? Perhaps, but if I do have seizures, I will know how to cope, will know what medicines I can and cannot take, and won't have to run off to the Emergency Room.

I have started working part-time for a job that sells cleaning and beauty products that are non-toxic and do not contain harmful chemicals, which I've learned can also cause toxins in the body. I still get fatigued and have speech issues in the evening. I still need naps during the day, and I have gained over thirty pounds since this all began. I need to have the lesion monitored, but at least I know that it wasn't the lesion that caused most of the side effects. I have a way to go, but I thank God daily for all of the things that I can do now that I couldn't do before.

I hope to use all that I learned through this terrible ordeal to help others learn and cope with aphasia, apraxia, dystonia, a genetic condition, and non-epileptic seizures. Life is a journey, and it has its ups and downs. I've found that the best way to bring your life back up is to help others up on your way.

61

Person with PNES, UK

The material in this chapter is based on extracts from a personal journal.

AUGUST 19TH, 2015

Okay, it's Wednesday. A week ago, at 1.30 p.m., I started not feeling very well, feeling weakness in my limbs and breathing slowing down, lightheaded and dizzy, with my five-year-old daughter asking if I was okay. I asked her to call for my middle son, who is eleven years old, who wanted to ring his dad, but I told him not to bother daddy, ring granny for me because at this point I was struggling to lift my arms and I didn't think that I was going to stay awake. I managed to speak to my granny and say can you come, then the shaking started in my right hand and my speech started slurring, and I thought I was bloody dying. I knew I had to stay awake for my children and told my middle son to call my eldest son to come down to take my daughter away from the situation, and at this point came the terrifying experience of my speech not coming out. I told my eldest son, who at this point was crying, to dial 999 [the emergency number in the UK] and to man up. To which he did. Sounds harsh doesn't it, but even at that point, I knew I had to get him to focus; otherwise, he would freak out and that wouldn't have been any good. I managed to ask my middle son to ring his nanny to come and get them, and at this point, my granny arrived. I don't lose consciousness, I was awake and fully aware of what was happening, and this frightens me even more because I am scared shitless as I don't know what is going on and I think that my body is giving up on me. What I didn't realize is that, last Wednesday I was suffering from non-epileptic seizures and probably saying what the hell is that, well add it to my many medical problems.

I spent a few days in the hospital, pumped with anti-epileptic drugs that didn't work. I had an EEG and ended up on the Stroke Ward (not sure why). Finally,

I got diagnosed with non-epileptic attack disorder by a junior doctor; apparently, the top consultant had reviewed my case. I was given a brief description of what it was, a website to visit, and told to go see my general practitioner and perhaps see a psychiatrist!!!!! My response was at the time "I'm doing this to myself" to which the consultant replied no of course not, are you stressed, depressed or suffer with anxiety . . . MY WORLD JUST CRASHED!!!!!

I have suffered (on and off) with anxiety for years. Anxiety to somebody who doesn't suffer with it, well they find it hard to understand why someone would panic and put barriers up to go to their local shops or why you would have thoughts that you're not worthy, that nobody likes you, not wanting to go out with even your friends and constantly pushing yourself into these situations. Doubting yourself because you're not sure if you will make everyone happy around you. But this is me, this is who I've been since I can remember!!!! Unfortunately, what this has meant to me is now I've got to a point that my body can't take the anxiety and pressure that I'm putting on my mind all of the time, and it's been decided that I sort myself out by manifesting in non-epileptic fits and tremors.

Now I have another journey to climb, and it's my fault, I should have told someone how I was feeling, the battles I was fighting in particular that I thought my husband was going to leave because I'm also losing my eyesight and I have endometriosis, which makes my life difficult with pain management. I have three beautiful and amazing children and work full-time, which has also added pressures that I've not shared with my husband. Not to mention my childhood, when I was constantly at the hands of bullies and family break up and the pressure that put me under; I didn't cope too well with it. My husband, though, he is the most amazing man I have met because since this has happened to me, he has been by my side and listened to me. He has given me the support that I need to know I can once again beat this. He has been understanding and has kept a watchful eye over me and given me the space and the encouragement that I have needed.

Am I crazy? That is a question that I've asked since the consultant told me what was happening to me. I'd probably say yes, but according to a website I've been reading, apparently I'm not; however, the problem I have is that there is no medication to treat this condition. I'm going to rely on myself to sort it out. So I've decided that I'm going to document my journey. Maybe it could be therapeutic too, better out than in, as they say.

I went to the general practitioner as soon as I could with my husband by my side, desperately trying to fight another nasty seizure. The general practitioner was great and really honest. "I don't know what this is; any advice from the Consultant, any hand over notes?"

"No," was my reply, "they think it could be linked to anxiety, stress or depression."

"Okay, let's put you on an anti-depressant."

My husband mentions that the consultant did mention counseling. He didn't mention a psychiatrist, but I didn't either. "Bloody hell, do I really need a psychiatrist?" The only problem is there is a huge waiting list for counselling. "Okay, we will go private." General practitioner says let me find a private counselor that can help and who understands the condition. Two days later, the general practitioner rings to say the private counselors want up twenty-five hundred pounds for ten weeks. So he has managed to prioritize me with the surgery counselor, and that day I get a phone call with a date for my first session that week.

Thank goodness for that, I might actually get some answers. I've read the website a hundred times, and I need to fully understand this condition.

AUGUST 26TH, 2015

I'm going to attempt to cook a meal tonight because I've had a pretty good day today. So let's see. To be honest, the first three days were spent in the hospital with me basically feeling that if I lay down and went to sleep, I wouldn't wake up.

It also consisted of me being exhausted because of the constant seizures, but I did have some fun in the hospital as an old lady opposite me kept me entertained, at one point telling me I was split bitch for trying to help her, which at the time made me laugh. She kept trying to escape and put her belongings in other people's drawers, but she seemed like a lonely, old lady who was reeling from the attention of the nursing staff. Nobody came to visit her either, which was sad. She put her two fingers up to the nursing staff and poked her tongue out behind their backs, but to be honest, the ones she did that to needed it. She mentioned that she and her husband had been married fifty-nine years before he died two weeks before their sixtieth wedding anniversary, which I thought was sad but also lovely that she still thought about him. At that point, I thought I don't think I'm going to see that with my husband. I genuinely believed that I wasn't coming out of the hospital. But as tests started coming back—CT scan, EEG—as normal, I thought that it was going to perhaps be okay, but what the hell was going on with me?

When they said that I could come home on the Friday, I was relieved and terrified over what lay ahead of me and my family. I was anxious about what the kids would be like and how upset they had been and how I had worried them. I didn't know if everyone would see me as a freak or as my eldest said to me, "You're bonkers." My middle son just hugged me, and my daughter the same.

AUGUST 27TH, 2015

Whereas yesterday I had a really good day, hardly any shaking in comparison to other days, today is not so good! Didn't sleep after having pain in my right ear all night, still hurting today, dreamed loads, and woken by the shakes. Let's just say I've woken up pretty miserable, and the weather outside reflects my mood as it is absolutely hammering down outside. I wish I could sleep!!!! I'm thinking about all sorts, the kids, the house, school, work . . . Today I text my husband saying, "why f****** me?" That's the way I feel today. I'm angry and feeling rather sorry for myself even though the anger just isn't coming out. I haven't coped very well with the kids today, only little bits of arguing and deficiency, but I feel I can't tackle it. I feel so alone but very much loved. I feel like a freak and I'm not in control of myself or my life. Got to ring the general practitioner today to find out about counseling, and I'm hoping this will pick up my mood, but today I feel like I can't be bothered. I didn't even want to get out of bed, what is wrong with me when there is so much pain and suffering going on in the world at the moment? All those refugees struggling for their lives, and I'm having stupid tremors and seizures because I'm anxious, how can I be so selfish, I'm so lucky for what I have but yet I throw it back into everyone's faces. Everyone who cares about me. I'm not dying, I have a happy home life, wonderful kids and husband. I'm happy. So why am I so like this, what the f**k is wrong with me!!!! In my head there is no reasoning, in my head there seems to be no reality, I'm ungrateful!!!! I'm trying hard to turn the positivity back on, yesterday was good, I felt a little more like me, why today do I feel so down in the dumps?

SEPTEMBER 1ST, 2015

Okay, today I am feeling much better, don't know what's changed, but not shaking as much either. The doctor confirmed that I have an appointment with the counselor on Thursday next week, which I am really pleased about. I know it's not going to cure me, but it's the right direction. I've kept thinking I'm going to be back in work next week, but I think I need to be realistic. So I need to sort this out with the trustees so I know that I'll get paid. I'll feel better then.

I had a couple of bad days but also had a couple of good days. I've decided to keep a list of things that make me feel anxious to see if I can identify triggers. Today we've been to the beach, which was nice. My daughter enjoyed herself. I felt really light-headed all day and used my stress ball and managed to keep them at bay. Just had a slight one, which I controlled. I think that maybe my husband is getting frustrated with me, which I can understand, but I am trying. It felt like my heart was banging in my chest the whole time, I wasn't relaxed, but then I'm not sure how to relax and I suppose this is what I have to learn over the next few weeks. I'm hoping to get this under control as soon as possible but not sure how we can afford for me to go part-time, though, with my son going skiing and my other son wanting to go away too with the school. Anyway, at least I'm functioning, and I need to work through this.

SEPTEMBER 2ND, 2015

Okay, a really good day today. Feeling like me too. Still feeling anxious, but not any major shakes, little ones but not anything else, so a good day all around. Had a bad one in the night but don't mind that. Feeling really good today as if I can really beat this, I am very much worried about money, though, when I drop days etc., but I know I can get through this. I feel like a normal human being today, which is wonderful.

SEPTEMBER 7TH, 2015

Okay, been an okay day. So I'm good, getting there. Small seizures this afternoon because I was tired I think. Going to have a lesson on my sewing machine just to get the basics; it's been a long time since I've sewn. I'm excited. Going in to work Wednesday, and I'm excited about that too. My memory is not very good at the moment, I keep forgetting the simplest of things, I don't know why - it is frustrating me as I used to have an amazing memory. I'm also going to take my daughter to breakfast club tomorrow up at the school. I haven't done that since I was diagnosed because I haven't been able to. Got counselling tomorrow, too. My husband is going to take me to a spa; I'm excited about that too. I'm positive and am happy.

SEPTEMBER 8TH, 2015

Another good day! Went to the shops with my mother-in-law and sister-in-law. I coped really well, also had food out. I'm really proud of myself. I can't BELIEVE I did it!

I also took my daughter to breakfast club . . . one step at a time, but I'm doing it . . . I am doing it, it was lovely, I didn't realize how much I had missed our walk to school.

A couple of seizures tonight, but to be honest, I'm not surprised as I have done a lot today. Going into work tomorrow too for the first time; I'm nervous but also excited. I need to get back to normal . . .

AUGUST 19TH, 2016

It's been a year since these early days of diagnosis. I still continue to have my seizures . . . they are up and down, I can have a month of small, not-too-violent seizures . . . and then I have a month of violent, hurtful seizures, my whole body vibrates and I'm conscious, I think; however, my neurologist seems to think that I'm not fully conscious through watching my videos. Yes, that's right—I went to a private neurologist. I'm working bloody hard to make sure that I am able to live a normal life as much as I possibly can, alongside my eyesight deteriorating. I have a really good consultant, and I now have my pain under control. I have applied for a guide dog and been accepted after months of meetings and training so I can become independent and feel safe to get out and about. I do regular meditation, good enough diary, paid for private counseling after funding from the National Health Service finished, do yoga regularly, and working toward mindfulness. More importantly, I am working hard to change my thought process and put myself first, which is an alien concept to me. I am still working four days a week, and everyone is helping to manage the home. The seizures are really manageable at the moment, and it's gone well. We are going on holiday in a week, and I'm looking forward to that. I have found a private neurology company, I have had help, and that's why I've seen a private neurologist to get a referral into the non-epileptic attack disorder clinic that is running. I was quite cross when I found out that there was a non-epileptic attack disorder clinic as I have lost a whole year of accessing neurophysiologist support. I am really clear that I may not ever be able to get rid of these non-epileptic seizures, but I can definitely give it a good go or reduce them to such a manageable point. I'm on the waiting list, I have four months to wait.

OCTOBER 31ST, 2016

So here I am still waiting for the non-epileptic attack disorder clinic appointment. Everything has been off the rails lately; my seizures are just as violent as they were at the start of this journey. I wake up constantly tired; my motivation is failing. My general practitioner says that the only medical option left is a relaxant. I don't want to take them, and my general practitioner is not keen too. I think I'm depressed, which I know is different to anxiety. So after a long discussion with my husband, I'm going back to counseling, and I've found a cognitive behavioral therapy counselor and she has worked with non-epileptic attack disorder. Thank God!!!! Don't have to explain the damn condition. I'm hurting myself with these seizures now, and they are changing. Whereas I always knew when they were coming on, the odd one is catching me out and I fall over. My hands in particular are killing me, and I'm still trying to keep doing everything. I have had a lot of stress at work—as the Manager, I am responsible for everything, and we nearly ran out of cash to pay everyone . . . I'm barely holding on and every month is struggle . . . I need a new job, but who is going to employ a person who has non-epileptic attack disorder, endometriosis, irritable bowel syndrome, oh and let's not forget, going blind?

Feeling sorry for myself . . . I am concerned how non-epileptic attack disorder is affecting not just me but my whole family. This can't be a good situation for the kids or my husband. I'm trying to show them all that I am coping and I'm getting through this, but my motivation is lacking somewhat, and I'm really tired, really tired. My body can't take much more, I don't think. However, after recapping and reading my first couple of days, I can't believe that I was back in work four weeks after it happened and that I still go out for meals, go to cinema, go on holidays.

When I read other people stories of non-epileptic attack disorder, in comparison I am doing really well, and I'm trying not to let the non-epileptic attack disorder take away me and become a victim of this condition. Like I've done with my other conditions. I think trying to carry on and have a life that is happy and learning to live with this condition is the only way to maybe hope that one day they will stop. I really think that at the moment I perhaps maybe need to feel down so I can climb back up, and I've been through so much in the last year and a half and I'm looking forward to review these pages one day and hopefully I will be saying that they have gone or reduced to a minimum, maybe once a week . . . That would be amazing instead of daily . . .

62

Mother Whose Daughter Has PNES, UK

My daughter is fourteen and in Year 10 at a girl's grammar school (academically selective state school). She's very tall for her age (always has been, rather than suddenly shooting up), athletically slim, and very physically strong. A keen athlete, she loves all sports but particularly enjoys field hockey, horse riding, cricket, and street dance, and has represented school, club, and county at some sports. She had excellent health up to January 2015, and had all the usual childhood vaccinations. She is very short-sighted [near-sighted] for a child, which deteriorated rapidly between the ages of seven and ten, but everyone on both sides of the family are short-sighted, her father is very short-sighted, and she very much takes after her dad physically. She eats sensibly and healthily, isn't picky, and takes lots of water. She has a good group of mates, is comfortably in the middle academically (the staff say the best place to be as the top performers are always stressing about maintaining it and the bottom ones are worried they'll be kicked out), and we've checked all her online and social media activity and found nothing to worry about. There is no boy stuff either, and everything at home, with me and her dad, with her sister, jobs, money, etc. is all good. The school personnel are very surprised and said she was the last kid they expected to have any issues to deal with.

The first two weeks of January 2015 were very busy. My daughter has always wanted to cram as much activity into her days as possible, and also she got a dental brace fitted to her top teeth and started her period (without any drama). She was performing at a local theatre in *Grease* and so had some late performance nights and rehearsals, but still did her usual dance classes and horse riding. I did call time on the cricket and hockey, worried she'd be overtired. She then had a five-day residential Outward Bound trip with her school in Wales. She loved the trip, which included rock climbing and abseiling [rappelling] etc. and running into the North Sea on a freezing cold January day! After she returned, she had a bath on the Saturday evening and felt very faint. I put it down to exhaustion and possibly dehydration.

She had a good sleep, a big breakfast, and lots to drink, but on Sunday morning, she fainted again and we couldn't really bring her round, she just kept fainting. The paramedics came, and she was admitted to hospital for three days. She had an MRI, which was clear. Her blood pressure and heart rate were monitored (and continue to be), and there is no difference in them whether she faints, when she is lying down, sitting, standing, or walking. We were told to go home and wait for it to pass soon, probably in a couple of weeks—it was "pseudoseizures," and no further help or explanation was given.

For the next two months, she was fainting for forty seconds to two minutes about every ten minutes, sometimes every five minutes, and couldn't walk un-aided or attend school. I had to take an extended leave of absence from work. When she had an episode, there was usually no, or very little, warning, and she would slump forward but be "straight back in the room" when she came round. Slowly, it improved to once an hour, then by Easter she was walking again and only having one episode a day. We hoped it would soon be all over. We had some sporadic contact with the Child and Adolescent Mental Health Services, she had some sessions with a social worker, but it has taken her a long time to build up trust. My daughter also learned quite quickly to tell the social worker and any medical staff what she thought they'd want to hear, to avoid difficult conversations and through boredom of being asked the same questions time and again. We had two check-ups with the epilepsy consultant, who just shouted at her to get up and told us not to catch her. So she fell. This got worse again after a few weeks; she was back to hourly faints for a couple of months, and had a carer sitting with her all the time in school. Then it improved a lot over the summer and in September. However, the faints left a legacy of migraines and severe headaches in their place. Since October 2015, her situation has got much worse again. She is wiped out by migraines and at the moment is fainting every fifteen to thirty minutes and is off school. She also has hallucinations—about people, who are occasionally menacing. There are usually two to five of these people in the room with her, but generally she finds them friendly. She is very private about them. She is sen-sitive to light and loud noise, and can "see" the sound rolling up the walls if she's in a busy, noisy room with loud acoustics. Occasionally, she loses her sight completely thirty seconds before she faints. Sometimes people's faces go strange colors before she goes. She says her head feels like it's being squeezed and is too heavy for her body to hold up. She feels sick but rarely actually vomits. Very oc-casionally, she drops to the floor suddenly, without losing consciousness, and just says her legs have stopped working. Occasionally, she says she can still hear us talking, but she can't move or open her eyes. Sometimes she knows she will faint; mostly there is no warning. She has never wet herself during an episode. Her eyes seem to be moving under her closed lids, and her face can twitch—sometimes people mistakenly think she's laughing and it's fake. Occasionally, her breathing gets very heavy, like she's dreaming, she's being chased or struggling for breath, and she'll come round as she catches her breath. The faints can happen when we are walking, sitting at the table chatting and eating, watching the television, in the car, in a lesson, in the shower, lying down resting, literally at any time. She is incredibly pale when the condition is worse, and on bad days is a strange grey/green tinge, with yellow around the eyes. Her hands and feet are very cold on bad days, whereas before she was my hot-water-bottle kid, always warm. People will often comment to me (not in front of her) how dreadfully ill she looks; the physical toll is very evident. When things are bad, she doesn't want to get out of bed or do anything. She will cry and sob and curl up on the floor if I try to get her to leave her room. She sometimes bangs her head on the wall or doorframe. We've had some horrendous scenes—the main advice we were given was to "not allow her to be an invalid and get her in school, keep her routine," which is impossible at times and also a mistake sometimes as I'd take her in after several hours of negotiation only to collect her thirty minutes later. We really were left to just get on with it, and I chose to permanently leave work to be there for her. She struggles to sleep when the condition is bad—in fact, she often falls out of bed if she has an episode in bed, but also wakes up throughout the night and calls for me to settle her.

Some small things were discovered—hypermobility, an innocent heart murmur, low blood pressure. When things first improved in July 2015, we'd removed her brace on the advice of both a homeopath we'd taken her too and a chiropractor. It seemed she might have had a strong reaction or the hypermobility meant she reacted more to the pressure in her head from the brace. It did always worsen after it was tightened. But that didn't explain why it returned with a vengeance in October 2015 and has stayed with us. She was so happy that September, back to normal for a while, everything good at school with her mates, back on the hockey team, successful audition for a dance show but doing much less than before. After a few months with a lack of support, it returned. I called the consultant who said, "Stop thinking in linear medical terms," and couldn't explain any further when I said I didn't understand that and it didn't help. The episodes changed in December 2015 so that when she fainted, it sounded like she was choking or fighting hard to breathe; sometimes she went blue. The school personnel, who have been fantastically supportive, said they couldn't be responsible for her. In despair, we went to the Accident and Emergency Department, where a doctor finally sat us down and explained what hadn't been explained to us for the whole year—it was a mental health condition called non-epileptic attack disorder, but because we were being seen by Child and Adolescent Mental Health Services, we couldn't be seen by anyone else, despite the fact that the current treatment doesn't appear to be working. I know it seems ridiculous as we'd been seen by Child and Adolescent Mental Health Services, but no one had ever explained clearly the condition was a mental health issue. We now could see how it had been alluded to in other meetings, but no one had ever used those words before or clearly spelled it out. She's also had a few sessions with an ac- upuncturist earlier in 2016, I followed all of the clinical advice, to try and ease the migraines and headaches, which seem to be helping. All the school staff, counselors, and many of the medical staff can't believe how mature and resilient she has been with coping with it, but now it's come back, she's getting worn down, and missing out on so much normal teenage life and fun.

Currently, she is back in school full-time and only faints once or twice a week. But she does get incredibly low. It can be hard to determine what's normal mood swings for a fourteen-year-old girl and what is a warning sign—her mood swings are extreme. There has been wider fall-out from the last two years of course; now we come up for air, you can see the social damage it's done. In many ways, she's more mature than her peers because of everything she's been through, especially the dark times; conversely, in other ways, she's stuck where she was two years ago. It makes her a difficult person to be friends with sometimes, and she has pushed friends away and some also got a kind of "carer fatigue," I believe. I also think she's missed so much school, or been on a reduced timetable, that she's become de-institutionalized from school in a way, and really does struggle with the every day, every week thing now. I know no child loves going in, but they're kind of resigned to it and it's part of routine, but she really fights it after so much time out.

She is very angry that this has happened to her and worries that it will never fully go away, which is of course terrifying when you're fourteen. We do feel abandoned and left to just get on with it and muddle through.

63

Person with Epilepsy and PNES, UK

A LETTER TO MY SEIZURES

For more than sixteen years, I was me. Okay, there were things that I struggled with, but I just carried on as best I could because I thought that everyone experienced what I experienced. But then when I turned sixteen, I had my first tonic-clonic seizure during the day. Following a few more (which always occurred at a meal time), I was eventually referred to a neurologist who diagnosed me with epilepsy. Suddenly I was no longer me; I had become "the epileptic." This first happened when I was in the hospital for tests to confirm my epilepsy, I overheard a nurse referring to me as the epileptic in bed X; I confronted her about this saying that I had a name and would she kindly afford me the courtesy of using my name. Of course, that didn't make me popular, but at the time, I didn't care. My life had been turned upside down, and no one really cared about me; they only cared about you (the seizures). Because of you, I had suddenly ceased to be a human being; instead, I had become a walking medical condition. Upon your arrival, suddenly so many doors were slammed in my face. Because of you, I was continuously being told what I couldn't do; no one ever thought to say but you can still do such and such. I resented the fact that once you arrived, you invaded my every waking moment. I was made to take medications that didn't really help to quiet you down but instead made me feel really ill. One of the medications completely changed my personality, making me really angry and irritable, but because it quieted you down a little, I was ignored and made to continue with it until it no longer had any effect on you. You managed to drive a wedge between my family and me. I was the eldest and had always been trusted to look after my siblings, but now I was no longer trusted to do that. Instead, my every move was watched by the family; it was like living in a glass box. I hated it and became increasingly withdrawn and moody, and that too was deemed wrong by all concerned. I couldn't do right for doing wrong. If I joined in and you butted in, that was wrong as I was seen as inconveniencing everyone and even frightening people, but if I withdrew, then that was wrong. Eventually I rebelled and did everything I could to assert my independence. I took up sports that I really shouldn't have done as you still weren't under control, and I cycled for miles each day. But it was my way of trying to run away from you, but it didn't work as everywhere I went you were sure to follow. No one ever took the time to sit me down and talk to me about what I was experiencing; all they were interested in was when you were at your most visible, showing yourself as a tonic-clonic seizure. I continued to experience brief absences and other partial seizures, but I was ignorant as to what they were. After trying several medications, I eventually found one that made you disappear, or at least I thought it did as I went for a long period without any tonic-clonic seizures. I grabbed this opportunity with open arms and applied to train as a nurse. I enjoyed the work and qualified and was good at my job, but unfortunately, I was attacked by a patient and seriously injured. My injury was treated though not cured, and it remains a problem to this day. Suddenly my world became really confusing, and I honestly thought I was going mad. I was so distressed by what was going on that I ventured to tell people, but I was simply labeled as attention seeking, which couldn't have been further from the truth as the worse it became, the more I withdrew as I was embarrassed to let others see what was going on. I was sent from one psychiatrist to another and was treated atrociously; I wasn't believed and was told in no uncertain terms that I was simply attention seeking. Eventually I was sent to see another consultant who before I'd even sat down said, "You're not going mad; I think I know what's going on, and I can help you." Tears streamed down my face, finally I had someone who believed in me, and it turns out that it was you and not me who was playing up. This consultant had an excellent registrar [a doctor who is still in training] who spent hours with me, and gradually we pieced together what was going on. It was you that was creating all this havoc in my life and not me. Had you been a physical entity, I'm sure I'd have killed you once I found out what was happening. Suddenly all the little strange things that had been happening to me all my life made sense. I had thought that either everyone experienced them or that they were simply a part of me, but no, it was you, you little ****, continually interrupting my life and making it difficult. As a youngster, I'd found ways around what was happening, but it transpires that by doing that, I was simply allowing you to take over my life more and more. Gradually the registrar and I put together a list of all my seizure types and auras, and once I knew what I was up against, it was easier to deal with. Things should have then progressed, but because we'd worked out that it was you that was causing my problems, I got the sack, which also meant that I lost the only doctor who'd ever truly believed me and been on my side as I was seeing him privately and insurance was part of my salary. But of course when I was dismissed the insurance stopped. I was then caught off guard, and once again you stepped in with glee to make my life a misery. You don't always show yourself in ways that are described in neurological textbooks, and so when after several years of trying to get a replacement neurologist I finally found one who would see me, they didn't believe me despite the EEG test showing clearly that you were actually there. You think you're so ruddy clever, being able to elude treatment for all those years, but I'm telling you now you're not; it was simply that no one had the thought to ask what was happening to me or what I was experiencing. Had they done so when I was younger, perhaps I wouldn't have gone on to develop dissociative seizures. I only developed those because of the way you made the medical profession treat me. You ruined my life, not because I had to carry you around with me but because no one had the intelligence to seek you out in all your different disguises.

But finally I got the help that I needed, not from an epilepsy specialist or even a doctor, but simply from a therapist. She gave me back the dignity, confidence, and self-esteem that you had robbed me of over the years. Gradually, as they returned, I was able to see you for what you were, a ruddy nuisance and certainly not my fault or of my making. You fed on my stress and anxiety, but as I slowly managed to reduce those, I found that I was slowly starving you out of existence. Okay, you've not gone by any stretch of the imagination, neither are the dissociative seizures, but you no longer phase me or make me panic. I can take you for what you are, a pain in the butt. You don't have a life of your own; I mean, I can exist without you, but you can't exist without me. I no longer panic when you show yourself as a partial seizure, and as a result I can cope much better. It also means I'm not feeding you, and so one seizure doesn't turn into two. By doing my best to ignore you, you seem to lose interest and go away, at least for the time being. So you see, with the right professional help, I've learned how to put you in your place. You've not gone, but you no longer terrorize and frighten me like you used to. In fact, on many occasions, I'm now able to see the funny side of some of the things you make me do. Okay, at the time, I don't find it funny, especially if you place me in danger, but looking back I'm now able to laugh at the absurdity of your behavior. You're not clever, simply a nasty little bully who gets their kicks out of menacing innocent people and ruining their lives. I can't get back the many, many years you've stolen, but I'm determined to make the most of the time that I've got left, and you're not going to spoil it for me. Basically, you can either fit in with me (pardon the pun), or you can naff off [go away]. I'm not wasting any more time pandering to your needs, and instead, I'm going to put myself first for a change. Your behavior over the years has been atrocious, and you should be ashamed of yourself. But on the positive side, you've made me far more aware of the difficulties others experience for whatever reason. You've also made me a far more compassionate and caring nurse, and I've tried to continue to be compassionate and caring even since leaving nursing. I've learned patience and acceptance and that what has happened is in the past and we can't go back. And that's where I'd like to leave you, but I know that that's not possible, and so instead, until you start behaving, I will do my best to ignore you and get on with my life as best I can. Finally, I would like to say that in the past, you may have won many of the battles, but you certainly haven't won the war. So think on that, my dysfunctional pain in the butt.

Yours without love or affection,

Me.

64

Person with PNES, USA

I first passed out at work back in 2013. It was Valentine's Day, and we were very busy at work. I work for a small animal clinic, and I am the office manager. We had several emergency surgeries, so I had sent all the staff to the back to help the doctors. I was holding down three phone lines and helping everyone that was walking in the door. I remember feeling funny and dizzy. The first thing I remember is my vision got very blurry. I bent down to file a record and passed out, or what I thought at the time was passing out. The doctor walked by and saw me lying unconscious on the floor. They were going to call for an ambulance, but I came to and said to just call my husband. When my husband got to the clinic, I still wasn't feeling normal, so I had him take me to the doctor's office that was just down the street from my work. I passed out two more times on the way there.

When we got to the doctor's office, they brought a wheelchair out to help me in. When inside, I fainted again. At this time my blood pressure dropped, and the doctor called for an ambulance to take me to the hospital. I was completely aware of all the conversations, but I couldn't respond. It was like I was paralyzed. After I got to the Emergency Room, they ran all sorts of tests. They first thought it was my heart. All tests were normal. I took a couple weeks off from work and rested. Well, what I call resting. I painted my entire first floor. I only had one speed; rest wasn't something I knew how to do. Long story short, fast forward a year, and these episodes continued to happen, but they were worse. I would twitch, mostly on my right side. I was referred to a neurologist who diagnosed me with epilepsy.

That was a very rough year because I didn't have epilepsy; the anti-seizure medications made me a mess. I couldn't function; I had reaction after reaction to the medication and was sleeping an average of twenty hours a day. I went to this from being very active; I had worked forty hours a week, was a mother of three active teenagers, wife, and volunteered at my church every week. My life was in total chaos. My husband was so worried, and so was everyone that knew me. I wasn't even the same person. All this time, the episodes were getting worse and were happening daily. I had to take a leave of absence from work.

My neurologist finally sent me to a specialist after nine months. I spent a week in the hospital for a video-EEG. I was lucky; I had several episodes while I was there, and they diagnosed with me psychogenic non-epileptic seizures. I had done a lot of research on my own while waiting to get in to see the specialist. I was happy to have a diagnosis, but I was also devastated. There was no magic pill or surgery that would help me. I knew I would have to do some very hard work to deal with it and hopefully overcome it. I had a cousin that has the same condition, and she is pretty much home bound. She doesn't work, and she is in her thirties.

Over the last few years with all my health problems, it has been a very difficult time for me. As I had to face my abuse from my past, I felt very unworthy to pray and unworthy of love from my Heavenly Father. I have forced myself to continue to read, pray, and attend my church services. It hasn't been easy; I think my anxiety gets the best of me at times. But one thing that never changes is my constant love for my Heavenly Father and Savior. It's hard to explain to someone that isn't Christian, but this knowledge is so real, it's almost tangible. I know deep down inside that I am never alone, that I am loved. As I forgive others, my heart is softened and the barrier that I have placed, notice that I said I have placed, is lifted.

When it comes to many things in life, it has so much to do with our attitude and our desire to overcome. Life happens, and unfair things are going to happen to all of us. We can either learn from them and grow, or we can give up and feel sorry for ourselves and live like a lonely victim for the rest of our lives. I decided a long time ago to be a survivor, and I think it's my faith that helps me with this. I feel like everything happens for a reason, some because of the bad decisions of others, or our own bad decisions, or just because it's our destiny. Either way, it can be overcome. My values teach me to love unconditionally and to look at everyone as a child of God. They all have great potential; some are just lost and need more compassion than others. I feel like that often; I pray for compassion for all my shortcomings, especially as a mother. I hope that I can teach my children that life is worth all the struggles, that it is meant to be enjoyed, not just endure. Some days enduring is okay, but then we need to brush ourselves off and put a smile on our face and really live. No matter what happens, it's going to be okay; it is my spiritual beliefs that gave me that knowledge.

Someday I will be strong again, but even if I never overcome this, it will still be okay. I still make a difference in my own life and the lives of many others. I will continue to fight and be kind to all. I will learn from my bad days and will truly enjoy my good days. I've learned that I do much better when I write my feelings down; I need to share and not keep everything bottled up inside. As the years have gone on and the challenges have continued to come, the one thing that I've learned is that you have to take time for yourself. When I rest, relax, and nourish my brain and body, the condition has less control of my life. It still is a presence in my life more often than I would like. I've learned that it won't ever go away, but I've learned how to manage it. I think that is the biggest revelation that I've had this far. People with diabetes have to learn to control their diet and manage their disease; people with depression need to learn how to manage triggers and what they need to do to cope. So I have psychogenic non-epileptic seizures and it's not an easy disease to have, but it's mine to learn to cope with and persevere.

65

Person with Epilepsy and PNES, Kenya

I hated the fact that no doctor could tell me exactly what was wrong for three years. I was taking medicines and still getting the seizures, and nobody sensed that there was something amiss as the medicine was supposed to help me get better. I have received therapy for more than three years, but I was only told that I had non-epileptic seizures less than six months ago. At least once a month or bimonthly, I would experience them. I hate the side effects of the drugs, and when doctors are really not sure of what they are treating, you then become a guinea pig.

It started in 2011. One Saturday, I was in bed upstairs, and my three kids were playing downstairs. I couldn't feel my feet or move them. I picked up the phone and called my mum and my boyfriend, who was not in. I tried to call my mum a second time; however, when I tried to speak, words could not come out, and I was stammering and making funny noises. I was alone in my room, and I remember crying and wondering what was happening. I could not alert the nanny or kids, so I just lay there waiting for either my mum or my boyfriend, whoever reached me first. My boyfriend arrived first, and all I could do was stare. I could not talk or move. He carried me downstairs to the car and drove like a madman to the hospital.

By the time I reached there, I was jerking and screaming because my head hurt so badly, I kept telling them to cut it off. They had to sedate me because the jerking came, then the headaches. I made funny noises when I jerked my feet, hands, and head, and then had a terrible headache, and then I blacked out. I could not move any part of my body during the blackout, but I was conscious and could hear all that was said. I felt numb. The doctors ran all the tests and found nothing. I was hospitalized for two weeks, and all manner of doctors came to check on my case. I could speak in a slurry manner, but I couldn't stand or walk. I did all manner of tests, and I remember feeling sad and isolated. Nobody was telling me what was wrong, and all the tests came out clean. I had an MRI that came out clean. One brain surgeon said I have tissue scaring on the left side of the brain that was causing the seizures. I did not know what that was.

I was sent home with drugs that made me drowsy and with the following instructions: Do not drink alcohol, drive, eat chocolate, drink coffee, or swim. At one point, I remember thinking my life was over; I even asked if I could have sex. I stayed home for one month, being bathed, fed, and driven to hospital for more drugs that made me more of a zombie. I felt depressed, afraid, and angry. At one point, I refused to take the medicine and to go back to work; I quit life. I wasn't myself anymore, and I hated it. I remember a time I did not sleep for two straight nights. My brain was not just shutting down. I even got a date-rape drug, and the person who gave it to me was very shocked, for hours later I was still wide awake even after taking it. I was taken to hospital only to be given more drugs and different types of injections to make me sleep. I took the drugs faithfully, but the seizures still came back. The doctors kept changing the drugs and experimenting, and I kept wondering—if I'm on drugs, then why are the seizures still coming back?

How has it affected my life? I went from a self-assured, happy-go-lucky girl full of life to a scared person who doubted herself. The drugs made me add weight, and my face got ugly pimples. At work, when I fell in my office, I was so embarrassed and had to stay home for a week so that my body would come back to normal because every time I got a seizure, my whole system would shut down and the medicines would shut it down even further. I loved going dancing and partying, but that stopped because I felt like I would fall at any time. When I fell, I never lost consciousness, but every limb in my body would stop working and bad headaches followed. After some time, I learned how to tell that the seizures were about to come—I would start to tear for no reason (and it's not because I was crying), then I would smell something that other people around me did not smell. Then I felt dizzy or woozy and would fall or faint; then the jerking would start from my stomach, legs, and hands and then to my head. I would jerk and make funny noises, then stop and black out or go limp. I could hear all the commotion going on around me of people trying to remove my clothes, blow air, do first aid, but I couldn't speak or react. I would feel nauseated and even vomit. When I came to, I would have splitting headaches, and I was too weak to move. Driving myself was not allowed, but I refused the doctor's orders as they were robbing me of my life. It was embarrassing to wake up to my colleagues staring at you, and I constantly apologized for scaring them. My boyfriend had to deal with being called to pick me up or stay with me in hospital for long hours because my mum lives far away. My kids did not understand and cried when I got an episode in the house. My youngest daughter still runs and hides under the bed far away from me every time I'm sick or recovering. After some time, I realized I forgot things; some memories no longer exist. I would meet relatives or friends and ask what is so-and-so doing, and people would look at me funny because the person died a long time ago. As a result, I stopped asking about their friends, mums, or brothers. When my boss gave me instructions, I would forget, and so I learned to carry a notebook and jot down word for word all what was said. I worked in a digital advertising agency, which meant sleepless nights or working long hours. Getting sickly all the time was not funny; I was in charge of managing sixteen people. My doctor recommended that I quit my job because it was too demanding and stressful, but I wondered who would feed my kids. He said the seizures were triggered by stress, lack of sleep, and not eating enough.

I recently met a doctor who told me that I have non-epileptic seizures; I was very excited that I am not sick and that I do not need to take different types of medicines. But now I have to learn about these non-epileptic seizures. But I'm happy once again.

66

Person with PNES, UK

I am currently twenty-four years old. My diagnosis of non-epileptic attack disorder was made in January 2009 at the age of seventeen, or eighteen months after my very first seizure. Although I was grateful to finally have a diagnosis for what was happening to my body, it didn't make things any easier. I was constantly in and out of Accident and Emergency as no one around me, except my closest family members, knew what was happening to me, and due to not knowing any of my triggers or warning signs, I ended up with numerous injuries from falling down, including broken ribs, dislocated shoulders, fractured coccyx and pelvis, along with burns and scalds. Ambulance crews and hospital staff up and down the country had never heard of this condition before, and I was told ninety percent of the time that I was making it up and faking my seizures: "How is it possible for you to be having something called a seizure if you're not epileptic?" This was very infuriating and led me further down the path of depression. I lost friends due to them not understanding what was happening, or why it was happening, as they didn't know how to deal with the episodes and stopped inviting me out, which at the age of eighteen was very difficult. I struggled with my education. Every exam I sat, I would seize, but with an extra year at college, I finally passed all my A levels and made it to university to study sociology. I ended up deferring due to ill health halfway through my second year. I have yet to go back as life and health got in the way, but I am determined to finish my course.

My neurologist told me that non-epileptic attack disorder isn't generally treated with anti-seizure medication like epilepsy is, and that there was nothing to take as such to help with my seizures. I was put on an anti-depressant to try and manage my mood and hopefully reduce my seizures. As there was no medication to be offered, I was told about cognitive behavioral therapy, which I attended on and off over a three-year period. Although it was an extremely difficult time for me as I was uncovering some darkness that I had suppressed from childhood, I cannot thank my therapist enough as she helped me not only come to terms with my seizures, but also helped me understand why I was having them, where they had potentially come from, and the possible original stressor as to why they suddenly started at the age of seventeen in the middle of my first English literature A-level exam and not beforehand.

In 2013, I spent the month of October in a specialist Institute of Neurology. I had daily appointments with a cognitive behavioral therapist, a physiotherapist, and an occupational therapist. Although at the time it felt like it was a waste of time and I wasn't learning anything, the impact made a difference when I got home. I had made friends with eight other people of various ages from both sexes and from various backgrounds and walks of life, but we all had one thing in common—these seizures—and simply knowing you're not alone made a big difference to me. I was taught grounding techniques, which I still use. I learned to recognize warning signs and identified some triggers. I remember wondering why on earth would I need an occupational therapist for a seizure disorder, but she is the one that has made a lasting impact. She helped me do simple day-to-day things again, the things that people take for granted, like being able to take public transport, go into crowded or busy places, or even sit comfortably in a coffee shop—generally, going out and socializing without worrying about potentially dropping to the floor. It really is the simplest of things that make a difference in life.

In 2014, I got my first home with my partner, a lovely bungalow (no stairs as I tended to fall down them a lot and break something either me or a hoover [vacuum] usually). Life has changed a lot since then. I have additional support where I have carers come in up to twenty-four hours a day if needed so that I am not alone at any given time if my partner is at work. Although I know this is for the best as I have on many occasions nearly drowned from seizing in the bathtub, it is still extremely annoying not being able to have a bath in peace.

I have vacant seizures where I seem to be in my own world, and although I appear awake, I'm not actually there, staring off into the distance or appearing to be ignoring someone and just looking through them. I have drop seizures where I can be walking down the street in mid-conversation with somebody and just hit the floor. I have seizures with twitching and eye rolling, violent shaking, and different tics. Some physical, some vocal, also dystonic seizures where I literally go "ironing board" still and arc backward. My heels can touch the back of my head in one of these episodes, which other than it being painful I wouldn't mind so much, but if I try and touch my head to my feet consciously, it's impossible.

On July 4, 2015, I remember finding it amusing that something like this could only happen to me on Independence Day, I had a really bad seizure while eating, and when I came round, I had no feeling or sensation in the lower part of my body. I couldn't move my legs, feet, or toes and couldn't walk or tell (as I had no sensation) if I needed the toilet. I ended up in a wheelchair for the next eight months. With the help of a physiotherapist and hydrotherapy, I eventually got back on my feet using walking aids. I can still remember my excitement the day I managed (with a lot of concentration) to move my big toe. I felt like I had just climbed Mount Everest. Over the course of time in a wheelchair, I was informed that the muscle weakness and loss of sensation were just another part of the seizure disorder, and I was informed that I had functional neurological disorder and that it was all part of the same thing.

Over the years of living with this condition (along with the numerous breaks and injuries), I have dealt with temporary paralysis in different limbs and temporarily lost different senses, but taking on a positive outlook, I learned sign language for when I lost my hearing. I have lost my eyesight and my ability to talk properly—it comes out sounding strange even though in my head I think I'm saying something properly or just completely forget what I'm talking about. And often pre-seizure, I can smell odd smells or get a horrible taste in my mouth.

It has been many difficult years, but my seizures have become part of my daily life and the lives of my friends and family. I try my hardest not to let this condition get in the way of living my life. I try to focus on what I can do, not what I can't, for I am someone who has a condition, I am not defined by this condition.

For the past eight years, my seizures would average out at least one a day, though I could go a week without one and then have seven all at once. However, I am currently thirty-one weeks pregnant with my first baby, due in February 2017, and since around June 2016, which would have put me roughly four weeks pregnant, my seizures have decreased to approximately three a week. I am not sure as to why but have presumed it's something to do with the hormonal changes my body is currently going through. I am worried how motherhood will change me, and how my seizures will affect the life of my partner and myself with a new baby, but I will not let this condition win. I will be a mum, a partner, and a friend . . . not "that girl who has them weird seizures."

Thank you for taking the time to read my personal account of living with this condition. Here is a favorite saying of mine about this condition and how I explain it to other people: "Some people save their moves for the dance floor, but my body prefers to rock out ANYTIME."

67

Person with PNES, USA

To my knowledge, my seizures and blackouts began after a fall/accident. I began having neurological symptoms afterward, including vertigo, facial numbness, and severe headaches, and I would be unable to account for long periods of time. For example, several times I was driving on trips approximately two or three hours from where I live, and then I'd suddenly wind up somewhere and not know where I was or how I got there. Another episode, I went to a take-out restaurant and waited for my order. But then suddenly, the employees there explained that I got up from my seat, walked toward the door, and dropped my keys in the water glass of a customer eating there. I remembered nothing about it. Suddenly I was standing at the door and not knowing how I got there and began looking for my keys. The workers there had called the police, who questioned me, and then brought in an Emergency Medical Technician after asking me EVERYTHING to determine that I was lucid and that I was fine. But yet they asked me about the incident with my keys, and I remembered nothing about it. That went on for months.

Several months later, I fell over in the parking lot of a restaurant with a grand mal seizure and was taken by ambulance to the hospital where I had no recollection of it, or of having bit half my tongue off, or that my oldest son had picked me up and taken me home. I had not sought help for the blackouts until the grand mal seizure. I would convince myself that they never happened or that I might have taken some medication that was making me have side effects. I certainly had some narcotic-type medications that could have. However, the truth (which I didn't want to admit) is that I had not taken any medication or had it in my system at the time of the blackouts or grand mal seizures.

I went to my next neurological appointment and told him about the grand mal seizure. He seemed agitated and told me that now we have to start all over again with the tests. Then he told me that I could not drive for the next few months.

The fall was in August 2014, and within a few months, I began to have problems functioning, which was so bad that I could not do my work; I lost all my jobs as a landscaper because I was unable to design; my brain wouldn't function. One of the clients that I had worked with for several years told me that I was not the same person they had known; she reported to me that I would be walking around in the yard and just staring up into space. She asked me, "Didn't you say you had a head injury?" But I still hadn't put the two together. Even though I wasn't able to function, I would keep convincing myself that no way that fall made me not be functional and I would just snap out of it. Another client said the same thing to me—that I was not the same person they had known for many years. But not knowing what was wrong, they both just accused me of probably being high on medications, but not able to pinpoint exactly what it was. By that time, I was taking narcotic medications, but it was after I was no longer able to work because I started to have so much pain in my muscles and joints and the feeling like I was being electrocuted in different parts of my body. But also, I would feel like I was just shaking from the inside out. Losing large amounts of time, even in my own house, and winding up somewhere and not knowing how I got there. My mom came to visit; she and my dad live three hours away from me. I thought it was to help me so that I could get rest and start to feel better, but two days after she got there, a police officer came to my front door to escort me to a mental institution.

My mom was trying to have me committed there. I was examined by their clinicians, psychiatrists, and medical doctors, who found that I showed no signs of being psychotic, and I was let go after one day. Since I wasn't able to drive and there were strained relationships with my mom after that, my dad drove a seven-hour round trip in one day to take me to my next neurological appointment. The neurologist told me and my dad, for the first time after all of my tests, that the diagnosis was functional neurological disease. He also told my dad that I was not crazy. He further told my dad that if he wanted him to write a referral to a psychiatrist that he would, but further explained that it would be a waste of time since I wasn't crazy, and that all they could do would be to regulate medication. I was given a new referral every time I went to the neurologist. By the time that I had researched about the department that I was referred to in order to prepare for following through on the referral, my neurologist changed to another referral and told me to just forget that one, he didn't feel like that was going to be able to help me.

Next, I am following up with a neurologist for a second opinion with a psychiatrist. Temporarily, the only thing that works is anti-epileptic medication and a pain reliever for the pain. These have seemed to help the blackouts, but I have not made anything but small trips away from home after the neurologist cleared me to drive. I don't think that the answer is in the pill, but right now, it is helping me until I can find something that is. I have been unable to work; my dad has been helping me pay some bills until the point he has no money left. And at this point, I feel helpless and don't know what to do. I'm so confused and feel like I need a simple starting point with a regulated, well-organized treatment plan. I feel like I'm being bounced all over the place, and I was already confused and in mental fog. I need help. My primary symptoms have brought in secondary symptoms of depression, anxiety, and feeling paralyzed like a deer in headlights in my own home. I just feel hopeless. I hope that I will find something that helps and more awareness with neurologists to know how to treat patients like me.

68

Person with PNES, the Netherlands

My wife was scared of my non-epileptic seizures at first, but after doing some research, she feels more sure of what to do and what not to do when they happen. I don't see my friends often as they still tend to "freak out." And colleagues? I do not have any more because I am unable to work.

My wife and doctor have both reacted very well to my seizures. At the hospital, the reaction is normal because of their job. Therapists are still wondering if it is real.

The seizures have had an impact on my independence and financial stability, my worklife and career. I no longer have a job, and I am still fighting to get some welfare.

At first, it was hard, but now, after a year, I see my seizures as part of me. I am a changed man, and if others cannot see that, or understand, then that is their loss.

At the beginning, I just had to find out what was happening to me by asking for the results of the tests done by my doctor. When I saw the results, I called the hospital for more information. They just told me that I had my diagnosis and that was it for them. Wanna know more? Just look it up. And that was that. And so began my crusade of finding out as much as possible.

At first, I was scared out of my mind, but after a lot of research and understanding, it is all a lot better. The seizures are just now a part of me.

When I feel a seizure is coming on, I use a weighted blanket to prevent it from happening. When I am too late, then I will also use the weighted blanket so that the seizure stops—in my case, within seconds. For when I have a seizure, a weighted blanket is a lifesaver. And by using an herbal oil on an almost daily basis, I went from fifteen seizures a day to just one!!

Hope that this might be of any help to you.

69

Person with PNES, New Zealand

I am not sure when it started; I just I know that it started. I was a teenager when I first had an episode that led me not to be able to walk. It sucked. It really did. My memory is blurry of that time, but I do remember being in the back seat of the car, while we were driving to the hospital, as I was unable to move. They thought I was drunk, but because I had been born with hydrocephalus, they erred on the side of caution. Thank God for the hydrocephalus; I hate to think how they would have treated me had I not had that previous condition. What is it with medical staff? They seem to all treat patients as criminals, except instead of innocent until proven guilty, it's the other way around. I remember that they didn't do much. My CT scans were fine, so were my x-rays. My parents didn't come and see me; I think they thought it was drink- or drug-related. I was a rebel, but I needed my parents.

It was the next year that I started getting these paralysis episodes more often. At the time, I was living away from home for the first time, and I lived with what ended up being my future husband, now ex. He took it very seriously, given that I would cry at how very frightening it was to not be able to move. I remember thinking that it must be in my head, that of course I can move; then I would slightly move a toe if I fought as hard as I could. I didn't know about seizures back then. After a shunt revision, it seemed to go right for a couple of years at least. I wasn't quite ever the same, though. I would be exhausted after days at university and scolded myself for being just too lazy. Little did I know, I wasn't at all.

I struggled through my university degree and started to work. My health was declining, but I had no idea why, and it was so gradual that I thought it was in my head. Until I struggled to even complete a ten-hour working week, that is. I could do it, but it was a struggle. My now husband and I went to the neurosurgeons first. They told me that my shunt was okay and sent me on my way. I went to my general practitioner and tried to make sense of it all. I didn't realize that my paralysis and tiredness were due to seizures of the absence kind, and I was unaware that the holes in my memory were due to the same. My ex-husband was getting more and more frustrated, all but calling me lazy and pushing me to do more. I tried. I really did. I never felt like I was good enough for him anyway, and I had been struggling with depression and anxiety for so long I blamed it on that, not him.

It wasn't until we ended our relationship that the first "shakey" seizures started. I think it was around about the time I was with my new partner, and I attributed them to the drugs I was taking. I was put on anti-epileptic drugs to "stabilize" my moods, when it just triggered worse seizures in me and more often. There are great big holes in my memory about that time. I was the rock in everyone's lives, and now I couldn't be that rock. I ended up with no one. Eventually I had to move back home, and that was the hardest thing for me to do given that my parents are emotionally abusive at times. I remember seeing the look on my mother's face and how much it looked like she thought that I had failed, yet she didn't seem surprised. I was, though; I expected my parents to be concerned and loving.

Almost six months later, I moved into my own place, and I started having a feeling like there are worms wiggling through my brain. It was the worst kind of torture, and I tried taking pills to make it stop, I even smoked some weed. I couldn't stop it, and I ended up in a massive panic attack because of it and passing out. My landlord called an ambulance. The hospital didn't have a lot to say about it, just that I was okay and to go home. That feeling of worms in my head started plaguing me on and off for months. Sometimes pain killers and muscle relaxants would help; other times I would be tortured for many hours, not being able to make it stop and feeling exhausted at the end. If I am honest, I wanted to take my own life more than once during that time. This was my life, which was horrible: my husband was no longer my husband, my parents were unsupportive, I had lost most of my friends, and I lived on my own in a little flat with a bossy landlady. I tried to get out, but life was hard. I struggled to walk down the driveway at that point.

70

Person with PNES, UK

I have been having seizures since I was eighteen years old. I had my first on a gap year [a year between leaving school and starting university in which the student typically travels or works] in Australia, and it is by far the scariest experience of my life. I couldn't understand what had happened or why. The camp nurse where I was working told me she thought I might have epilepsy and to go to my doctors when returning to England. I couldn't understand how my life could change so quickly. I then began to have them more frequently. I went from being extremely confident and outgoing to very introverted. I didn't want to leave the house, I lost my job, I lost friends, I couldn't afford the rent or bills, my life seemed to change within a year so drastically, and I couldn't understand what had happened. I even lost my university place. I was going to study to be a teacher, and at that time, for me to do that I needed to be clear of fits for two years. I became depressed. I was now having about five to six fits a day and was so scared of leaving the house. I was worried about having fits in public and what people might think about me; I was worried about crossing the road, people mugging me while unconscious, or worse. I became house bound. I remember once needing some milk while my partner was at work. I decided to walk to the shop at the end of the street. It took so much strength to even open the door to my flat. Then adrenaline kicked in, and I just started running, I ran and ran, straight past the shop, and kept going. I remember thinking, what am I doing? Stop running! When I did, I looked at my feet and I still had my slippers on. I ran back home and cried. I have never felt that low and never want to feel that way again.

Now my seizures are much more controlled, and I have a much better life. I don't feel that they control me anymore. I am a teacher and a mum, and I leave the house without concern (normally). But I am still very ashamed of my condition. I know people judge me, whether it be friends, work colleagues, or hospital staff. It can be very hard to explain what my condition is as most people immediately assume it's epilepsy, and when I explain it isn't, then they think that I am a freak or faking it. That is probably the worst thing about the condition. It's embarrassing. I know what they think because they will openly make comments or gestures in front of me about it.

I suffer with dissociative disorder after my seizures and will struggle to walk and speak. A lot of times, I get accused of being drunk, especially if I have been out and had a drink; this makes me wary of socializing in certain areas. I have been dragged off the floor by paramedics and told that they "have had enough of this!" because I was struggling to gain my balance on my feet. I have had bouncers beat up my boyfriend because they thought he'd dealt me drugs. I have had a previous boss tell me that when I am "tired," that's not an excuse not to be in work! I have a seizure medical identity card and a bracelet, and have even given my bosses information regarding my condition, but somehow these things are still overlooked. So now I find I make a joke of it; I call it "breakdancing!" That seems to be less scary, less of a big deal, and more manageable. The truth is it's easier to laugh it off than deal with the looks people give you, the fear in their eyes, or pity. It's easier to be blasé.

I have reached a point where I feel that my seizures are controlled. Last year, I only had three. That is major progress. But I don't work full-time and know that that will probably never happen as if I am too tired I am more susceptible to seizures. I have to cancel on friends regularly because I don't feel well; I don't want to risk ruining their night by being unwell while out. I have had to teach my son from an early age how to dial his dad and 999 [the emergency number in the UK]. I have to constantly be aware of my moods, feelings, and hormones. I had to give up driving. But at least I am not having five to six seizures a day; at least I can bring up my son and teach. That fills me with pride when I think about where I was and where I am now. I worry about people judging me as a mum, a teacher, and a friend because of this condition. In so many ways, I am so happy I have reached a point where I can live a semi-normal life. But I wish I could stop them completely. I wish I could work full-time, I wish my son didn't have to know what to do if mummy is ill, and I wish I could go out without worrying about what might happen and do my friends know what to do? I wish the condition wasn't so stereotyped.

I am grateful that I have good support and a good family, and a good group of friends and colleagues who don't judge me now and understand it. I think that is what makes it bearable. I try not to think about what if my seizures stopped; I have done that so many times and been so disheartened and destroyed when I had another. So now I just remind myself how far I have come, and take pride in that.

71

Mother of Person with PNES, UK

My daughter started to have seizures when she was eighteen and on gap year [a year between leaving school and starting university in which the student typically travels or works] before going to university. The seizures developed in intensity and frequency over several years and had a major impact on her life—both academic and personal—as well as on my life and, actually, on the whole family. I had some understanding of epilepsy (but had never witnessed a seizure) but had never heard of non-epileptic seizures. I was relieved when we were told it wasn't epilepsy (I was worried about the medication) but was left bewildered when given no further help—if it wasn't epilepsy, there was nothing that could be done! I took my daughter to the Epilepsy Society for a second opinion, which confirmed it wasn't epilepsy. We then looked into whatever we could think of that might help, such as nutrition, brainwave patterns, Irlen syndrome, and eventually heard about cognitive behavior therapy and a program being conducted at the hospital in the city. Fortunately, I was able to pursue these avenues in order to try and get the help that my daughter needed.

I found it difficult to deal with the actual seizures and with the dissociative behaviors afterward, such as difficulty walking and talking. She looked and sounded as if she had been drinking or taking drugs, and others obviously thought she had. It was awful to be woken in the middle of the night by the telephone call from one of her friends saying that they had called the paramedics because she had had several seizures and couldn't be brought round, then driving twenty miles in the early hours to meet her in Accident and Emergency and seeing staff still trying to bring her round. I was also called out of meetings at work to be told that she had been found unconscious in the corridor or toilet and the "CRASH" team had been called—her clothes cut off. Sometimes she was so deeply "out" that she did not even respond to pain. The medical view was clearly that these seizures were attention seeking—I was told by a medic not to let her see that I was upset because that would gratify her behavior. I remember telling the doctor what I thought of that, given that I had been up all night having met her in Accident and Emergency.

I was concerned that she was at risk when going out—she had passed out on buses (even been brought to the house by a bus driver late one night). She was frightened, and I was very worried about what could happen to her. She had to return to live with us as her relationship broke down, and I drove her to and from work and often had to turn around and return home with her because of a seizure. When she first went to the hospital for cognitive behavioral therapy, I had to accompany her as she wasn't safe on the trains—she even passed out in the Underground, and I had to get help from the staff to clear an escalator to get her up safely. Developing the confidence to travel on her own again became a major goal of her treatment, which she finally achieved. This enabled her to regain independence and her sense of self. My daughter had to forego her place at university—her ambitions were being taken away from her by this condition. But she persevered and reapplied to university a few years later. She experienced discrimination as the doctor carrying out her occupational health assessment was obviously ignorant of non-epileptic seizures. Thank Goodness I had accompanied her as she would not have felt able to challenge him on her own. We did it together. And with the help and support of her therapist, she gained her place at university.

I am proud to say that my daughter has completed her degree, is now a successful teacher, and is someone who will try to help others with non-epileptic attack disorder and is willing to stand up to prejudice. She is a devoted mum and has fought to access the help she needs at school. She still has seizures, less frequently, but she no longer lets them rule her life. She takes appropriate precautions to ensure her and her son's safety. I couldn't be more proud.

72

Person with PNES, Australia

The seizures that I experience are closely related to the posttraumatic stress disorder that I have from military service. So by monitoring and appropriately dealing with the issues arising from posttraumatic stress disorder, I can minimize the duration and violence of the seizures when they do occur.

73

Person with PNES, USA

I have been diagnosed with non-epileptic seizures since 2014. I received therapy for a full year. I was a seizure free for a year and a half, from June 2015 to December of 2016. My last seizure was thirty minutes ago. Every day, it varies how many I experience. Some days I can have up to twelve to fifteen. Sometimes I can have a little as three or four a day, which is the least amount of seizures. Sometimes I can't walk, which leaves me paralyzed. I also experience the inability to talk. I have memory lapses as well.

On top of the seizures, I am also diagnosed with post-traumatic stress disorder, anxiety, bipolar disorder, depression, and dissociative identity disorder. It greatly impacts and affects my life. I am actually disabled right now in every way possible. I cannot work; I actually had to quit my job last month because of the seizures. I cannot drive because of the seizures. They are unpredictable. Sometimes I get signs that a seizure is coming, like seeing lights or spots, but lately I have not been getting any signs. I have to actually move because I currently live in an upstairs apartment with my fiancé and I cannot get up and down the stairs, and when I go out, sometimes I have to use a wheelchair. I can barely get out of bed in the middle of the night, sometimes because I'm paralyzed from the seizures, and I have to literally drag myself to the bathroom.

This is my life. It is extremely hard and extremely difficult. The condition takes its toll along with the depression. But I am still hopeful. I hope that one day I will find a doctor or a group of doctors to help me, to help everyone fighting this condition that is common but leaves those affected by it feeling very much alone. I don't want anyone to go through this living hell. Thank you.

WAIT AND SEE

Please don't judge what I am about to say,
For this is something I go through each day.
Fluttering fast goes the lids of my eyes
And here I go once again, no surprise
My head slowly begins to nod up and down,
I am aware what's going on, I just can't make a sound.
My right arm begins to tremor and shake.
Then my body erupts, explodes, and quakes,
Violently I thrash and move all around
Unable to stop, my heart rate pounds.
Beating so hard and so fast,
When will this be over, how long will this last?
Then I stop and fear follows in place,
Terror etched all over my face.
For I am trapped from within a hell,
Forced to watch in my eternal prison cell.
All I want to do is run away,
In this state I do not wish to stay.
It feels like something has taken a hold,
Leaving me empty, a human mold
Of a person who I once used to be,
All I want is to be seizure free.
All I want is for the pain to go away,
And look to a brighter day.
I just want to not live in fear,
And no longer cry a river of tears.
I want to no longer carry these sorrows,
But instead have a happier tomorrow.
Sadly when I awake, it will be the same,
I know truly that the trauma is to blame.
What I need is help and support,
Not be turned away and cut short.
Stop calling this made up or fake,
For that is something I can no longer take.
I need these doctors to do more and care,
So that maybe when I go out, people won't stare.
I need my life back, I need to be free,
I know I have to hold on, just wait and see.

74

Person with PNES, UK

I was diagnosed with non-epileptic attacks in February 2014, although they started in October 2012. I have seizures every day, sometimes as many as six. It has gotten better; at the beginning I was having between twelve and twenty a day.

My seizures all started when I had septicemia. I was in the hospital when they started; the doctors didn't have a clue what was happening. The stroke doctors and cardiologists saw me, but they couldn't find anything, so I was sent home. It continued to get worse to the extent that my fiancé had to leave his full-time job to look after our kids and me.

My son is now eleven and my daughter five, but when this first started, he was seven and she was one. It has been unbelievably hard on my son because he remembers what I was like before all this, while my daughter doesn't. We don't go to that many places anymore, and I can't go and do all the fun things that we did before, like swimming, ice skating, and fun fairs (the flashing lights are a trigger). I went to a fun fair not long after these attacks first happened because at that point I didn't realize that flashing lights were a problem. As soon as the ride started, the strobe lights began, and almost immediately, I passed out. They wouldn't stop the ride, so my family had to stand there and watch me getting thrown about like a ragdoll. I severely damaged the muscle in my right leg, which still hurts now.

This condition has taken over my life, my fiancé's life, and my kid's life. We are scraping by on benefits. My partner was a bar manager, and I was seven weeks away from being a qualified nail technician and beauty therapist. Life was good, and then it just crumbled away. It takes a long time to accept that this is the way my life has to be now.

75

Person with PNES, UK

On September 16, 2015, I fell over in the street, hitting my head on the pavement really hard on the left-hand side of my face and breaking my right arm! My partner drove me to the hospital where I had x-rays of my face; they weren't sure if I had broken a cheekbone. It was confirmed that I had broken my arm, but my face was okay—bruised and cut but no broken bones. Thank God! I was sent home with a sling and a head injury leaflet!

Then, on September 19, 2015, my right arm felt numb and funny. I got grumpy, and my headache got worse! I went back to the doctors on October 1 as I still was feeling dizzy; I was having bad headaches and buzzing in my ears! I was told it was depression and was prescribed an anti-depressant.

On October 25, 2015, I had a seizure in the night! I was semi-aware, and I filmed it on my phone. I again saw the doctor who said it wasn't epilepsy and asked me to film it again!

On November 1, 2015, I had another seizure, which was witnessed by my partner.

On November 2, 2015, I had about five seizures. My partner called NHS Direct [a telephone advice service operated by the National Health Service], and they sent an ambulance. I had a big seizure, which I wasn't aware of! I was taken straight into resus ["resus," or the "trauma" area, is for seriously ill or injured patients with immediately life-threatening illnesses and injuries], where I continued to have seizures. I was given medication to stop the seizures. I had a CT scan that came back clear! Then I saw a lovely neurologist who said that I had confirmed post-concussion syndrome and thought I had epilepsy or non-epileptic attack disorder. I saw another neurologist. He witnessed a seizure and said it was non-epileptic attack disorder; I wasn't going mad and wasn't putting them on! He wrote to my doctor saying I had indeed got post-concussion syndrome. He booked an MRI scan and EEG, which thankfully all came back clear.

My seizures only happen at night around 3 a.m. to 6 a.m. My right arm is mainly affected; it shakes on its own. Sometimes I keep hitting myself in the face; I pull funny faces and make funny noises. Other times my whole body is affected like a grand mal seizure. Occasionally I have lost control of my bladder; it's really embarrassing! After a non-epileptic attack disorder seizure, I normally suffer from headache, brain fog, and fatigue, which is horrible. I feel awful for days after a seizure. My neurologist sent me to see a psychiatrist who knows about non-epileptic attack disorder, who then sent me to another psychiatrist for six weeks in August 2016. We worked on the trauma that I suffered in childhood, both physical and mental abuse as well as other trauma in my life, such as finding my grandma dead and having to deal with all stresses (e.g., calling the police, etc.) and post-traumatic stress, plus my partner works for himself and we have got serious money problems as he doesn't work that much, and the real strain of family life—we have two teenage kids.

My seizures are about twice a month, maybe more depending on my stress levels or if I have overdone things. My friend said that I should contact a charity for help as I still suffer from headaches, brain fog, fatigue, and I have trouble with words—I have to really try to concentrate as it physically hurts my head. I don't like crowds as I can't filter out noise; lights make my eyes go funny—I get dizzy and forgetful. Anyhow, this lovely lady from the charity came to see me and said that not all brain injuries show up on MRIs or CT scans, especially months after the injury has happened. She suggested that I had a mild traumatic brain injury.

On November 19, 2015, my arm went numb and I became shouty and grumpy. I have met two other people with traumatic brain injuries and their symptoms are the same, if a little milder, but they don't have non-epileptic attack disorder seizures.

I feel like finally I am not putting this on; I am not putting this on for sympathy. I have an injury and non-epileptic attack disorder seizures. Some people still do not understand, including my general practitioner—I had to tell her that postconcussion syndrome and non-epileptic attack disorder seizures, these horrible conditions, have completely changed my life but I won't let them beat me!

I have good days and bad days. Finding people who understand you on Facebook support pages and other non-epileptic attack disorder awareness sites are great help, but I feel that people with non-epileptic attack disorder are not treated with respect and there is no help available as doctors aren't aware of the condition! People get accused of faking their seizures!

Non-epileptic seizures have completely changed my life—some days I barely get out of bed due to fatigue and pain all over my body! My memory is bad, but luckily family and friends are really supportive. Without them, I am sure I wouldn't be here to tell you how living with a traumatic brain injury and non-epileptic seizures is a complete nightmare. I joined support groups for functional neurological disorders and depression. I volunteer and I am admin on a depression awareness Facebook page, which has been a great help as I feel less useless doing something useful and helping others helps me! I found talking to people who are going through hell living with depression, non-epileptic attack disorder, or a traumatic brain injury is really helpful. Also, helping others with conditions that you are fighting every day has been really helpful as I feel so lonely. There's no other help or offer of advice. Non-epileptic attack disorder affects a lot people's lives day by day, but no one knows about it! You are told it's non-epileptic attack disorder seizures and just to deal with it by yourself, no medication; meanwhile, your life is in tatters and you find it hard to carry on! Oh, you are so lonely until you find others who suffer the same as you and realize that you're not mad or alone.

76

Person with PNES, UK

I've been having nonepileptic seizures for about five years, and for the past three years, they have been at least three times a week. They can range from just a mild seizure, where I can just collapse and then come around and need a little sleep, to collapsing and not knowing where I am or even remembering how to talk or move my arms and legs. I'm fully there when trying to move or talk, just nothing is happening, and it's terrifying. I'm just glad it only lasts between ten and fifteen minutes, even though it feels like longer. Sometimes I know when a seizure is coming on and I can just about tell my husband so he can hold me before I fall, but most of the time I have no clue it's about to happen.

It affects my day-to-day life constantly. I'm physically and emotionally weak all the time. Every seizure completely drains me, and just as I'm getting over one, I have another one. It's like a never-ending cycle. I struggle to do most things now—just walking to the toilet or kitchen drains me and I have to sit down for a little bit. I have a three-year-old daughter, and it's horrible to not always be able to take her for walks or play with her all the time, and she already knows what to do if I collapse with her. She shouts straight to her dad and tells him; if he can't hear her or if he is outside, she will grab my phone and phone him.

I got diagnosed with this condition in September 2015. I'm on a waiting list to see a specialist about these seizures, and she will help me to try and cope with them. But I have been waiting for over a year now, so I am just stuck in limbo trying to cope and just live my life as much as I can. I'm constantly paranoid about having a seizure when I'm out and about. My husband is my carer, I need supervision 24/7, and I wear a medical wristband just in case. My husband had to stop working to look after me. He is amazing and I don't know what I would do without him, but I always think I'm stopping him from living and it kills me. My daughter is literally the best. I don't think I would have coped if it wasn't for her and my husband; I doubt I would be here right now if it wasn't for them.

I am very lucky—the amount of times I have collapsed, I've had plenty of scares and had to go to hospital but have only had bruises/swelling and a broken finger, also a fracture in my jaw, but it could have been so much worse. I'm so grateful that I'm still here today trying to get better day-by-day.

77

Person with Epilepsy and PNES, UK

I don't like the word *nonepileptic* seizures; as soon as someone says the word *epileptic*, they think mental and crazy—this causes me more anxiety. To be honest, you are probably better off being classed as mental because you would get a lot more help.

All I want is my career back, where I am not being given these benefits. I want to pay my own way and have my own money.

The benefit system annoys and frustrates me. When I go, I am often told that I am "looking well," which can go against me. I am confused how I am supposed to look—burnt out, tired, washed out?

Getting all wound up is something that sets me off, when so much is going off in my head, trying to get everything right that you just go overboard. The key is to keep calm. Breathing is the main issue; when it is rapid, short, and shallow—this makes my mouth go dry. Breathing properly is key to not getting all wound up.

Non-epileptic seizures are not a case of using drugs. It is about working with that person. Volunteering and gaining employment has been a great help as I am not always thinking of me. It takes my mind off it.

I saw a psychiatrist some time ago. I feel that counseling is just not enough. I just find it all so frustrating to deal with. I need to learn to just relax.

The condition is not spoken about enough. More people need to know how to deal with it when someone has a seizure in public, such as on the bus. After I have blacked out, I want to know what I was doing or what happened, but instead, there is no one to talk to about it.

78

Person with Epilepsy and PNES, USA

It all began six months ago. I was walking my pup in my front yard early one morning mid-June, and I felt a tingling sensation run down my arm to the end of my fingertips. I thought it odd but continued on. I dropped my daughter off at school and was driving to work. I started to feel off; my eyes started to feel like they were bouncing. My hands gripped the steering wheel. It was all I could do to see the road. I was frozen. I remember I kept thinking how I needed to pull over before I passed out or I got into a wreck, but I couldn't. I couldn't move. I was stuck for what seemed like thirty minutes, but I'm sure it was only a few minutes.

This day changed my life; it was the start of something I never had even imagined could happen to me. I made an appointment, but this one-time event started to happen more frequently. A week later, my doctor immediately told me that it sounded like seizures and that I needed to be seen right away. I went in to see my neurologist who even though I had a concerned primary care physician requesting further testing smirked and said, "You are not having seizures." I left with nothing but more worry because I had no clue what was going on with me. The events were still increasing and my body was starting to lock when they happened. I was so confused. My family contacted my primary care physician as the episodes were up to six per day, and I was told to go to the Emergency Room. I was finally admitted, and even though there were no EEG findings, they wanted to do further investigations. One neurologist said that I had hypoglycemia and to buy an exercise bike and ride it every day. Another said you can't base a diagnosis of epilepsy off electroencephalograms because it could be deep in the brain. One clinician said psychogenic non-epileptic seizures right away, just because I was on a postpartum anti-depressant. The hospital was supposed to admit me for three to five days, but after one and a half, they saw nothing on the electroencephalogram and dismissed me with a diagnosis of psychogenic non-epileptic seizures. Finally, in December,

I was taken by ambulance to our local hospital, and they diagnosed epilepsy after seeing something on the electroencephalogram.

It has been such a horrible roller coaster. I lost my job over this, and the worst part is I cannot even look for work because there is no way I could work like this. Ever since the seizures started, they seem to have adapted or changed over time. I recently started having grand mal seizures, or what looks like them to my family. I have had as many as twenty-one in one day and have never had a day without one since they started. I can't go out in the sun or enjoy social events; it's completely insane. I went from full-time mom with a full-time job who rarely was home to someone who barely leaves the house and stays in the dark a lot. My kids also have to stay home more as I normally took them everywhere and I can no longer drive. They now watch me, like babysitters. It's awful. I hate the fact that I am no longer independent.

79

Person with PNES, UK

I have been having non-epileptic seizures since January 2016. It wasn't until November 2016 that a neurologist diagnosed me. This was after months of being in and out of hospitals, test after test, and being in around about thirty-five ambulances as no one could explain what was wrong with me. It was very scary.

When I have a non-epileptic seizure, I don't get any warnings, yet I will usually be sitting when it happens, but on a few occasions I have been standing. The first I know of this is waking up on the floor and feeling confused; it takes me a few minutes to realize what's happened. I will usually be sick or feel sick and very shaky. My heart is usually racing, and I will seem a bit in my own world for few moments (as others have noticed), and sometimes I will get body pain. It usually takes a good day or two to feel better. I will feel drained.

I had never heard about non-epileptic seizures before November 2016. I was scared when I was diagnosed. I felt alone, and I didn't know how to explain to people that after months of tests and hospital admissions, I finally have a diagnosis that I don't understand. Most days I wake up worrying, will it happen today? Will it be a bad one? And when it will happen?

80

Person with Epilepsy and PNES, UK

I started with non-epileptic attack disorder back in October 2009. It came out of the blue as I had never had one before. After being treated for epilepsy for two years, after an EEG and video recording, I was told that it was actually non-epileptic seizures. I was at the time having three to four seizures a week. They tried to wean me off my epilepsy medication and my fits went through the roof, so I was begrudgingly put back on them, which are also mood stabilizers, and the seizures settled down to my normal pattern. I was sent to see a psychologist and had weekly sessions with him for just less than two years, but this had no effect on my seizures at all. I have in the past had multiple daily seizures for as long as two or three weeks and then they settled again, but last May my seizures started being anything from three to six a day and I also started losing control of my bladder, which I hadn't done before, and now nine months later, they are still the same. I am so depressed. I do have a fantastic husband who is my full-time carer but have been virtually house-bound as after each seizure I have a banging headache and need to sleep. I have done more injuries to myself falling while having them, broken bones, cuts that needed stitching, and have a permanent bad back from the knocks.

This must be one of the least understood yet debilitating illnesses I know, and people (and even medical staff) really need to understand it better as I sometimes get the impression that when you try and explain it, people think you're making it up. I was on disability benefits until I came up for review, and I was awarded it when I was having three to four seizures a week and not wetting myself, but have had it refused this time when things are far, far worse. And we now have the extra stress of having to go to appeal; it's disgusting. Thank you for the chance to let me tell my life as it is.

81

Person with Epilepsy and PNES, UK

My seizures make me feel confused; I didn't and still do not understand why they happen. I have had them since I was seven years old. I never understood why I had to spend time in hospital as a child and why my mum and school were concerned. I also feel helpless, like I have no control. I have felt anxious, but having them for so long, I have had to adapt my life to manage them. I have encountered discrimination, misunderstanding and bullying in workplaces, and a lack of support in that environment; I have had to walk out of jobs that I have enjoyed not because of performance or attendance but because I have seizures.

My school years, although difficult due to my condition, were the most positive. My friends and teachers were fabulous and supportive, and I was never bullied at school because of it. I developed a positive attitude toward my condition and never let it wear me down or stop me from attempting things and living my life; it is only being an adult that I have experienced bullying, ignorance, and intolerance, which damaged my confidence and is currently making my new employment difficult to settle in. I hate the embarrassment that having a seizure causes, like wetting myself or talking gibberish or appearing drunk. The indignity of waking and seeing people around you and not be able to talk, not understanding what has happened. Why are you on the floor? Why does your head feel like it's going to explode? Why do people look frightened of you, like you're mad, abnormal, or just concerned?

My wife understands and accepts me; she's my rock who fills in gaps, my memory, an absence, or just keeps me safe. I couldn't manage without her. My family has been through hell with thirty years of my life taken by seizures. But I have deep frustration with my doctors, my diagnosis changes, I don't know what to think, it's not explained, so much time lost, I deserve better. I have post-traumatic stress disorder and as-yet-undiagnosed, high-functioning autistic traits, which are possibly compounding my post-traumatic stress disorder symptoms. The world feels alien to me, and my body doesn't feel my own. The post-traumatic stress disorder symptoms were caused after a horrific experience in my place of work due to my seizures.

I wake up every morning hoping it will just go away or I will feel different, everyday! But it's still there. I need to be alone sometimes, which affects my marriage, but how do I tell someone that everything I see around me looks unreal without sounding insane? My seizures she can understand; I am not sure she can understand this, so I pretend that I am okay, which is hard.

82

Person with PNES, UK

It was back in October 2014. I was at work when I felt acutely unwell. I thought I had gone into an irregular heart rhythm. My heart was jumping like in a *Tom and Jerry* cartoon. I remember saying to my boss, I think I've gone into atrial fibrillation [an abnormal heart rhythm], I don't feel very well; in fact, I don't feel very well at all. I remember her leading me into the gym, and my next recollection was being surrounded by paramedics and nurses. My chest was exposed; I had a defibrillator on my chest, oxygen in situ, and my colleagues in floods of tears. My eyes were apparently fixed and wide open, my pupils dilated, my heart rate 120, and my blood pressure 210/120. I was blue lighted [taken to hospital in an emergency vehicle] to our regional hospital and admitted to the Coronary Care Unit where all my colleagues work. It took another eleven months before I got my diagnosis. For four months, we went down the cardiology route; at one point, I was told I may have a pheochromocytoma [a tumor] on my kidney; I was even referred for a gynecological opinion in case it was hormonal. I had two more admissions to Accident and Emergency, one at a Christmas party for work and another while I was in the gym with the patients—I can remember feeling really vague as I walked out the gym, and my colleagues found me wandering in the corridor with a vacant look, dilated pupils, lip smacking, and only yes-and no-answers. Every episode I had would leave me with a splitting headache and absolute exhaustion.

It wasn't until I had my third admission to Emergency Department that my husband showed the consultant a video of me that he had taken. It looked like something out of a horror movie. My head was contorted, my pupils dilated, and I looked demented. He said that looks like absence seizures; you will feel like you've run a marathon and you've not even put your trainers on. Hallelujah, I could have kissed him, he was spot on, but then he hit me with you can't drive, you can't work, and you need to wait to see the neurologist. I have never felt such despair; everything I took for granted was taken away from me. I started having up to seven seizures a day. I developed a river-dancing left leg, which would take off on its own accord. I had Tourette's-like outbursts, which were so out of character. My daughter was doing her exams at school, she didn't want to be near me as it frightened her, my parents constantly babysat me, my son was eighteen, my husband stated he just wanted his wife back, we were due to go on a holiday of a lifetime, and we were celebrating our silver wedding anniversary, but that had to be cancelled as I was unable to go with an undiagnosed condition.

The first time I went on the bus on my own I had a seizure. I remember looking at the bus driver, but I couldn't remember where I lived or where I was going. Uncannily, about a month later, I was talking to a mutual friend, and he asked me why I wasn't at work. As I explained to him what happened to me, he said that he was the bus driver that day; he thought that I was drunk or had been taking drugs! I stood on my drive and just sobbed uncontrollably. I said to him never judge a book by its cover. This invisible illness is the most debilitating thing that I have ever experienced. My EEG, MRI, and CT scans were all negative, and my first reaction when I was told my diagnosis was, "Do you think I am making this up?" I was distraught. It wasn't until I watched a YouTube clip of a neurologist/psychiatrist and psychologist discussing that this condition can be triggered by past stress that you have not confronted or bypassed, and then something equally or more stressfully occurs and your body says I'm out of here. It all made sense to me then, as there had been and was still uncontrollable stress triggers within my personal/family life that I had no control over.

I was referred to a local psychologist who I had actually worked with and who told me that a high proportion of people with non-epileptic attack disorder had experienced abuse in early life and only ten percent was due to stress. I was in this ten percent, and as such, it proved difficult to access common cognitive behavioral therapy and other therapy methods as my stress was on-going. I was visualizing situations from my past nursing life, including a gentleman who had set fire to himself and a lady who stalked everyone who had looked after her deceased husband and accused them of murdering him! She even discovered where I lived and where my children went to school. My son had threatened to end his life and suggested we do it together. My once idyllic life was in tatters.

I remember one night I was home alone, the family was at the local football match, and I had had multiple seizures. I was exhausted with a splitting headache. I took painkillers and remember thinking I can't do this anymore. I'm going to take all these and my other medications. I knew where I was going to go, my medication would slow my heart rate to low levels, my blood pressure would drop, I would be pain free, and it would all be over. I now knew what being in crisis meant. Just at that time; a friend from work called me, and I made her talk to me for two hours. She begged me to allow her to come over, but she lived at the opposite side of the county. Without that call, I don't think I would be writing this today.

This debilitating, invisible illness makes you realize who your true friends are—just the smallest gestures mean so much. I forced myself to go out on a daily basis. I was going to the local bingo hall three times a week where I befriended two widows and a gentleman who had devoted his life to his mother who sadly had recently passed. I was constantly surrounded by people, but I was so lonely. My husband couldn't understand how I could possibly be lonely when I was never in. Those who suffer with this condition will know just what I mean. A true lifeline was the support groups on Facebook. I couldn't believe that there were so many people with the same symptoms and that numerous ones were nurses also. I have been in this profession for thirty years and had never heard of non-epileptic attack disorder. I have now been seizure free for six months. I'm pleased to report that I am back working twenty-eight hours a week, in a job that I love, with the most amazing group of nurses. I have always been barking [mad], but at least now I've got a diagnosis. I know I'm not the same vivacious girl I was, I can't juggle all the balls I once juggled, but I'm back, probably in part to the Equality Act 2010! Hope this helps someone.

83

Person with PNES, UK

I began to experience problems with dizziness and collapsing in August 2011. I was suffering dizzy spells daily, at multiple times every day, with intermittent collapses, where I would "be out of it" for a relatively short period of time. I would come round fully after sleeping for several hours. It wasn't until March 2015, when I had a particularly lengthy collapse and subsequently lost my short-term memory (couldn't remember my husband or my three children!), that I was admitted to a hospital overnight and later saw a neurologist, who diagnosed non-epileptic seizures. She spoke with me and my husband at length, and also with my daughter, who had been witness to a lot of my previous collapses, and filled in a lot of gaps that were previously unknown to a lot of us, such as limb jerking and twitching coupled with facial numbness that I had previously dismissed as nothing to do with anything.

I still experience daily dizziness but thankfully infrequent seizures (now we know what they are), although my recovery time and the effectiveness of my recovery seem to be taking longer recently. I get no warning whatsoever of an impending seizure, thus making life extremely difficult. I have to have a chaperone whenever I go out in case of a seizure. I can also no longer work or drive due to this condition. I am awaiting cognitive behavioral therapy, and although I have had no previous trauma or abject stress to deal with, my neurologist feels it is worth a try!

84

Husband of Person with PNES, UK

Put simply, I would like my wife back! Doctors have told us that this condition is not life-threatening, but it is life-affecting. Not just my wife's but the lives of our children, her mum's—who takes my wife out when I am at work and keeps an eye on her—and mine. This has had an effect on us all, not being able to enjoy life as it should be enjoyed, but with this shadow over us all the time.

85

Person with Epilepsy and PNES, UK

After several decades enduring a variety of what I was told were epileptic seizures (complex partial with secondary generalized), I was admitted to the hospital for four days of video-telemetry—that's when you have electrodes stuck to your scalp to measure electrical activity in the brain and two video cameras record every movement you make. This is done in a single-bedded side ward, away from prying eyes. The intention is to monitor and record seizures while matching them to the electrical activity in your brain during an episode and while doing ordinary activities like reading or talking. Your normal routine is deliberately disrupted, and medication is denied if necessary.

My first warning came at 1:50 a.m. during that first night without my medication. It was the old, familiar feeling of dread and fear rising from deep inside my abdomen like a porcupine coming from the inside, then spreading outward. I pressed my alarm button but nobody came, and I quickly went into the seizure. Terrified. Stiff and unable to move, except for rocking forward into an embryo position. I was gasping. No, almost roaring. Soon I began to hallucinate. At the join between the ceiling and the opposite wall, there appeared what seemed to be an army on the march. They were in shining clothes, almost like Roman legionaries of ancient times. But nothing was clear. This horde marched from right to left across my field of vision. Shields and spears. Silver, blue, yellow, always on the move, over hills and through valleys, driving me deeper into terror. Complete silence. Still nobody came. I suppose the staff had to let it all happen in order to record it. Eventually a young doctor arrived, and I was barely able to describe what I was experiencing, all the time gasping, clutching myself in that embryo position. The young doctor eventually recognized that the seizure was too profound to be allowed to continue and administered a sedative intravenously. It did not work, even when the dose was repeated. The colors in my hallucination became brighter, and my anguish intensified, until the doctor finally gave me a large shot of another sedative. I gradually became calm, and the visions disappeared. This episode had lasted five-and-a-half hours.

That was Day One, and many various seizures followed, all of them quite mild. At the beginning of Day Four, my consultant came into the room. He said, "I have some good news." But I did not believe him because he looked uncomfortable. "The seizures break down into two main groups," he continued. "The small ones are epilepsy, and the big ones are non-epileptic." It was an awful shock because it had taken me years to come to terms with having epilepsy, and now here was something new and big, which I did not really want to accept. I had read about dissociative seizures, but my consultant neurologist was insisting on calling them non-epileptic attack disorder. "Everybody will know what you mean when you say non-epileptic attack disorder," he explained. "It's what everybody is used to hearing."

Some months after my discharge from hospital, I had several sessions of talking therapy with an excellent psychologist who uncovered possible causes of the non-epileptic attack disorder. I'd had a dysfunctional childhood, living with a mother widowed by World War Two. She had grieved throughout my childhood and used her suffering to manipulate me with emotional blackmail. This led me to abuse alcohol for many years. After my first marriage broke up, my ex took the two kids to another country. She told me of her intentions during a phone call to my workplace. It was then that a colleague observed what I later identified as a non-epileptic seizure: non-epileptic attack disorder. The local hospital had always treated me very badly when I was admitted following seizures. Once, in the Medical Assessment Unit, I was left unattended while having a six-hour seizure, the kind I now know is non-epileptic attack disorder. On another occasion, the Accident and Emergency consultant made me leave while in the middle of a cluster of seizures. That had been the final straw, and I made an attempt at suicide by overdosing on sleeping pills. It failed, and I was admitted into a secure psychiatric unit for four weeks.

I remember having a non-epileptic attack disorder seizure in a subway station while on holiday. Nobody seemed to notice the hunched figure who was rooted to the spot and shaking with fear. Crowds of blurred figures hurried by in all directions. There was another time when a similar seizure started out of the blue when I was at home with a friend. Luckily, she was able to write down what she had observed for me to update my records. Sometimes, when alone, I have gripped the nearest solid surface for support and waited, terrified, until the seizure subsided. My psychologist and I came to the conclusion that my non-epileptic attack disorder is the result of a gradual buildup of all kinds of different stresses, many incidents resulting in that emotional overload. I have looked back over my life. The epilepsy was undiagnosed until I was forty years old, the non-epileptic attack disorder when I had turned sixty-six. My neurologist and psychologist now agree both conditions have been present most of my life. So what I had thought of as not quite achieving my potential can now be viewed as accomplishing much despite undiagnosed disabilities. I finished my career as Design Manager in a famous toy company; however, the downside of finally getting a definitive diagnosis was that I realized I am not the person I had previously thought. This caused an identity crisis that I battled with for several years. Another problem hidden from view, now thankfully resolved.

Now retired, my day starts when the doorbell rings at around 8:15 a.m. It's my carer, come to make sure I have a proper breakfast (my carers are among the few people who see me at my worst, which is grumpy and zombie-like and very wobbly). She will then leave me to finish eating. I tend to open my emails before taking my medications. It is a small encounter with the outside world and helps to stop me being insular. It's a necessary part of my strict routine of regular mealtimes and medication times. The side effects of the medications, and the exhaustion caused by the non-epileptic attack disorder and epilepsy, means I have to go back to bed and doze until my alarm rings at 11:00 a.m. Time for the second strong tea of the day, have a wash or a shower, and slowly become more conscious. By then it is time for lunch, which is a ready-meal heated in the microwave. I gave up cooking years ago, after some near-accidents involving absence seizures, kitchen equipment, and hot electric hobs [cooking stove]. During this period, I also kept accidentally throwing sharp objects because of involuntary jerking. It got to the stage where I reckoned I had better quit while I was ahead, rather than push my luck until the inevitable happened.

By the time I am fed, dressed, and have watched the lunchtime news on TV, it is approaching 2:00 p.m., when I will be ready to face the rest of the human race. I might go shopping, visit my favorite café to drink coffee while I read and write, or go to see a friend. I don't think people can see signs of the seizures often lurking near the surface, or of the identity crisis caused by the diagnosis of non-epileptic attack disorder. They certainly don't know of the exhaustion, or anxiety and depression, that accompany my impairments. Sooner than I would wish, it will be teatime and the TV news. Bedtime is usually 9:30 p.m., so any interesting TV programs have to be watched at a later date on the catch-up service. Once a month I go to a poetry workshop. We write a new poem every month during the academic year and have performed together. Some of us do a regular open-microphone spot at readings. Some have published poetry collections and won prizes.

Sometimes I recall with gratitude the time a man and woman came to my aid after I had a drop attack near a dangerous dual carriageway. To this day, I don't know if it was caused by epilepsy or non-epileptic attack disorder. It could have been either. But those kind-hearted souls remain as foggy images in my mind. I was too stunned to see them clearly. I would love to be able to thank them properly for calling an ambulance, and to let them know they are the only people ever to do me such a kindness. Some folks pretend seizures are not happening and hurry past, embarrassed. I also recall the taxi driver who spotted I was in trouble and took me straight to the local Accident and Emergency. He led me inside and handed me over to the first nurse he encountered. What a contrast between these good citizens and the Accident and Emergency consultant, a man who should have known better, who refused to believe I was having seizures, and who made me leave the hospital!

What I have learned: non-epileptic attack disorder has brought me through an invaluable learning process. I have always felt lonely and isolated. During my younger years, the loneliness was painful, and I could not understand the feeling. Now I see it as just the solitude I need in order to be me. I envied those people who were more successful in relationships. That said, I have a few outstanding friends who I love and who love me. You can't put a price on that. I'm comfortable with the person I have become and am enjoying some of the best times of my life. It might seem a strange thing to confess, now that I am pushing seventy-three, with the added limitations of age, but being forced to slow down and settle into the routine imposed by my disability has made me cherish each moment of every day, and to be thankful for every small achievement. I do feel at peace with this crazy world, although there is plenty needing change where non-epileptic attack disorder is concerned. I'm working on that. I look forward to the time when future generations will be diagnosed accurately and quickly, and receive respectful treatment whichever hospital they may be admitted to. Onward and upward, as they say.

CHOICE

A poem that shows how my philosophy for living took me toward the time of the diagnosis of non-epileptic attack disorder:

> It dawned on me.
> Only a lifetime's patience and respect
> might realize a worthy tilth.
> Nothing less could ever partner
> the momentary opening of Truth's Flower.
> Rather than crouch in the famine of a living lie
> I will await that moment in hope.

86

Person with Epilepsy and PNES, UK

I had the choice to stay overnight or go home. My whole body hurt, I could barely walk, and I felt like I had been at the gym for hours. I woke up one morning when I was twenty; I didn't feel well. I stood up and had a tonic-clonic seizure. I remember my partner being on the phone to the ambulance; at the time I thought he was speaking to me. The next thing I remember, I was in the ambulance, then at the hospital. They were not worried and said that it's quite common for people to have a one-off seizure. It was a week before my birthday. My family had bought me driving lessons, but the doctors said I would have to wait twelve months until I could apply again. I just wanted to go home and sleep. Little did I know that this was only the start of things to come.

Over time, I had more and more seizures. Eventually I was admitted to a neurology ward and put onto a thirty-six-hour EEG and video. Everything came back normal. This went on for the next few years. I had many more seizures, which started to take over my life. My family refused to believe it was epilepsy and thought that it was all in my head. I felt so alone and confused. I had to stop doing my college courses because they didn't have insurance with me having seizures. Feeling more and more alone, I just hid away.

I happened to have a seizure when one of my friends was taking my picture, so they accidently videoed the start of me having a tonic-clonic seizure. I spoke to the doctors, who agreed to send it to my consultant but who weren't actually that bothered. There was a problem with the file, though, and it wouldn't send, so they asked me to put it on a USB stick. I remember speaking to a friend the week before, crying, saying I'm going to die because I'm having so many seizures and nobody believed me. I had a two-year-old daughter; I was so scared I would put her at risk with the seizures. The day after I handed in the USB, my consultant phoned and asked me to come in the next day to the ward for another thirty-six-hour EEG. I had no support from my family; they agreed to take me to the hospital but just dropped me off outside with no help with all my bags. So they admitted me and hooked me up to the EEG, and a few hours later, I had a big tonic-clonic seizure on EEG and video. Finally, I got the diagnosis—I had epilepsy.

The next few days were a blur. Put on medication that made me feel awful, I continued to have seizures. I was in and out of the hospital with lots of bruised and broken bones. Been put on different sedatives, which knocked me out to the point that one time I was put into intensive care because my blood pressure crashed as I had had too much. I was sent to a specialist hospital for six weeks to monitor seizures and have another EEG and had cameras all over the ward. I wasn't allowed out of the building. I hated every minute. The staff treated me like I was a dog; they decided I was making everything up. I was told I do have epilepsy, then told I didn't, then told I had both (epilepsy and non-epileptic seizures), I was so confused. After four weeks, I was discharged, but I continued to have seizures.

My local Accident and Emergency made me feel like I was worthless. They said there was nothing wrong with me and I was to stop making seizures up. This got to the point my general practitioner had to write a letter saying I had a dual diagnosis. This didn't help. On one occasion I was screamed at, saying I don't have epilepsy and told to get out of the Accident and Emergency at three o'clock in the morning with only my pajamas on in the middle of winter; it was snowing heavily. There were no buses until five o'clock in the morning; eventually I got a lift home. This carried on for years. I had no life and told that I was selfish, that I had Munchausen syndrome. My family still didn't believe I have epilepsy despite a letter from my consultant saying I did. This caused a rift between me and my family, which was already strained. My partner at the time controlled me, put me down; this went on for years. It then came out he had been abusing our daughter. I was distraught, and my heart broke. I was also abused as a child, so it broke my heart because I vowed that my daughter would never go through what I had. I felt I had failed her. My family, friends, everybody took his side. It was hell. An old friend supported me and picked me up. Gave me the support I needed. We later went on to have a relationship, and I moved away from the town and had a fresh start. I knew nobody, but I needed to get away from all the hatred. This turned out to be the best decision of my life. After time, my daughter and I began to heal.

My seizures continued, and the same thing happened at the local Accident and Emergency. Any time I went in, I was spoken to like I was a piece of ****. On one occasion my general practitioner sent me to Accident and Emergency because I had hurt my back. I told the general practitioner I thought it was just a bruise; anyway, I ended up being blue lighted [taken to hospital in an emergency vehicle] to the hospital. I was in a lot of pain. I was brought to resus ["resus," or the "trauma" area, is for seriously ill or injured patients with immediately life-threatening illnesses and injuries]. They started drawing up medication, then one of the doctors noticed my face and refused to treat me, saying, "Oh, I know your story—get out of my Accident and Emergency." I wanted to know what was on my medical notes as to why I was always treated so badly, so I requested my medical records. Reading what doctors had written about me cut deep. My neurologist had written I made my seizures up, biting my tongue on purpose. Another doctor added Munchausen syndrome on my medical notes. I made an appointment with my general practitioner and challenged the diagnosis, stating as far as I am aware that doctor wasn't able to diagnose this as he is not trained to. My general practitioner agreed and took it off my file.

I was referred to a neurologist who specialized in non-epileptic attack disorder. On the first appointment, he asked what do I know about non-epileptic attack disorder. My reply was I don't really know. He then went on to say it's a very real thing and isn't made up and is just as hard as having epilepsy. This was the first time in nearly six years I felt someone finally believed me and wanted to help me. I felt a massive weight had been lifted. Since then I have gotten married and started treatment to try and help get me the help I needed. Regarding my daughter, the court case is coming up in the next few months, and I still continue to struggle with seizures as well as other medical conditions, but I have someone who believes me and wants to help. A relationship with someone who loved me for me and started healing some of the scars I have from my ex-partner.

Every day is a struggle. I'm housebound; I can't go out without somebody because if I have a seizure and somebody phones the ambulance, I will have to put up with the attitude of Accident and Emergency. I'm trying to move on with life, but it's still very hard.

87

Person with PNES, USA

I am forty-two years old, and I have experienced non-epileptic seizures off and on for most of my life. As a child, it was misdiagnosed; I was not on steady seizure medications until I was into my thirties. I have a hard time going places alone. My husband usually accompanies me. He can sometimes recognize the seizure activity and is able to intervene and help me stay in control and be safe. I have lost my driving license twice in the last few years. I have a hard time with anxiety when I'm going out because of the worries about what if I have a seizure. I normally don't go out alone. My biggest problem is the lack of information that doctors have with my condition, and their usual answer to any problem is more medication. Hopefully, this will help bring more awareness and education for doctors/neurologists.

88

Person with Epilepsy and PNES, UK

I have had seizures for over thirty years. I was first diagnosed with epilepsy, then about three or four years ago, the hospital carried out some videoing of my seizures as well as EEG tests to see where in the brain the seizures originated from. Because the neurologist couldn't see if my brain waves were being affected, the neurologist said that I had non-epileptic attack disorder and tried to explain that I could come off some of my medication as the seizures weren't epileptic in origin. But, I said, what if it made my seizures worse, what would happen about my job that I have? Because they couldn't give me a definite decision, I kept taking my medication.

Ever since I was diagnosed with seizures, since I was in my early twenties, I have been prescribed anti-epileptic medication. Now I am in my fifties, and I still have between two and three seizures per month, though most of them are quite small. After I have had a seizure, I feel very shattered [exhausted] and need to rest. When I have my seizure, it is like having nails hit into my head, and it hurts, and my face feels like it is moving, but I can't stop or control it. I can't stand up, and I will lose control of my legs and will be on the floor. I can feel my teeth chattering and smashing together. Eventually my teeth chattering will start to slow down, and at first I won't be able to get up, but after about ten minutes, I will be able to stand and just feel a bit out of it.

89

Person with Epilepsy and PNES, UK

I think my story has implications for children living around terrorism. In my country (Northern Ireland), it isn't acknowledged, but so many children do not get the help that they need. Terrorism creates an atmosphere of terror and anxiety, constantly worrying when is the next bomb going to explode. Children don't have the skills to control this fear and anger. When someone hurts them, they kick back, and I wanted a gun to kill these men hurting me. Children need a safe place where they can say, "Help me, I'm scared," and get the support that explains what's happening and gives them comfort without "cotton wooling" them as they need to adjust to the terror. It leaves them vulnerable to anyone, even dangerous people, who offer them the help they need. In the worst affected areas in Belfast, there are a high number of suicides in the young people.

My epilepsy developed and changed in reaction to my experiences of living around the troubles of terrorism. Only now, with the new diagnosis, do I understand it. When I was fourteen, I began "blacking out" during events and had spiritual experiences, such as visions and suddenly feeling as if I was in God's presence. My epileptic seizures started when I was twenty-one, but even the first ones were bizarre. I was on holiday with the family and came round in a hospital back home. I learned that three days prior I'd started having seizures, and they brought me back home. I didn't know how they had managed to move me, but I accepted it as a part of epilepsy. When I was ten years old, my younger sister started to have convulsions after an accident, so I knew about how the brain works, how convulsions are caused. And the family had coped with my sister for years, so it didn't upset us. I just had to learn how to adjust to this new illness. I was told I was drug resistant with uncontrolled epilepsy, which caused frequent seizures. I started having tonic-clonic seizures and what I finally called absence seizures, but they didn't all seem to follow the usual symptoms of epilepsy. Sometimes I'd come around badly affected, very disabled; other times I'd come around unaffected. My doctors wouldn't believe me or offer any explanation. I'd also click out for a minute or two, stop speaking, but I could still move and make hand gestures. The seizures suddenly changed to complex partial when I was forty-one. The absence type continued, but a new type of that also developed. I'd pass out, but I'd stay on my feet. It seemed as if I was in a trance; I would also come back around in a shorter time. I'd know that I was in the world, but I could make no sense of it for long or short times, unable to react to others but for all intents and purposes otherwise acting normally.

I grew up in a great, thriving, industrial city where we knew each other, there was plenty to do, and my sister and I could play outside. Three days in 1969, however, crashed my whole world. There were riots down our road, but I only felt tension in the air. Dad got more and more upset and finally lost his temper, strange as he was a quiet man, but I now know that he and his family had been badly affected by the violence. My parents didn't explain what was happening or try to protect us from what was going on, these strange loud noises that people called bombs, why were there soldiers arriving, what were those enormous heavy vehicles, why couldn't my sister and I go out as we used to. I soon learned about bombs; one morning we went for our usual shopping, but a bomb had gone off. I saw in a butcher's window a side of beef stabbed through with a large shard of glass. Oh, that's what bombs do. I had my first blackout during the next school year. My school was in an unaffected area, and a woman came in to talk about the troubles. I erupted in rage, how dare she, she hasn't had to dodge bullets, run for cover. The next thing I knew was "waking up" as the girls clapped at the end of the talk.

I'm still "stuck" in bomb mode as I often black out and don't know how I escaped. I had to learn how to live with the danger, the warning signs like security vehicles as our house was in a quiet area, but surrounded by working class estates who were already angry with our social injustices. I could be stranded, unable to move around the city as there might me bombs or riots. It was before mobile phones, so I couldn't find out what was happening or ask for help. We moved around the country; after three years we moved to the countryside where my dad ran an outdoors center. We soon learned that we were in what was called "bandit country," close to the border where the terrorists found sanctuary and made quick raids across the border. My sister and I went to the city for school and then settled there for work. I was studying to be a teacher. I didn't know how my epilepsy would develop, so I finished the course and tried some temporary jobs until I had a seizure in the classroom and scared the pupils. I had to leave and didn't know where else to go, but my pastor found me a job in a friend's office. However, having two bouts of flu and frequent seizures, I had to leave after a year. As I had no income and needed some care, I had to move back in with my parents. I was forced to stop driving because of the epilepsy. The public transport was an easy target, however, so it was cut back to the bare minimum. I spent two years in the countryside, virtually imprisoned, as we were deep in the country. There were no buses and my parents tried to help me by giving me lifts, but they were busy. I found that my training to cope with the conflict helped me adjust to this; I knew what to do in emergencies, how to look after myself if I was alone. I was frequently alone as well due to the social effects of the troubles—it was difficult to go out and meet people, plus most things like the cinemas had shut down. I was cut off from my friends when I moved to the country.

When I was thirty, we moved back to the city when my dad took ill with Alzheimer's. Finally, I took office qualifications when I was thirty-three and searched for work. There was still ignorance, fear, and stigma attached to epilepsy. In 1991, I was awarded Disability Living Allowance with a back payment sufficient enough that allowed me to go back to university; I later qualified at top of the class. The evening before my first day at the university, however, I suffered the worst bomb explosion and lost a very important day as I blacked out. The largest bomb ever used went off in a government building just opposite us. We were saved physically as we lived on a steep hill and the worst of the blast went over our heads. However, I had just gone into the kitchen when it exploded, something slammed into my back, and feeling the severity of the blast, I thought it was the ceiling falling and braced myself for death. When things settled, I was still alive and went into the living room where mum had been. I saw the chair I'd been using; it was pierced with a glass shard. This shocked me, and I made a remark to mum who told me off for making things up and we started to clean up. That's the last I remember until the next day as I stepped off a bus and "woke up" when I saw my damaged house. I had no idea where I had been, only that I was supposed to go to the university that morning—I found some notes that must have been given to me there. When I went back the next day, I knew nothing about the place, where rooms were, my tutors, etc.

After university, I couldn't get work, receiving what was really oral abuse at most interviews. I passed time by working as a volunteer, but I was usually left sitting at home with nothing to do. When my seizures changed, I decided that I could finally live on my own and moved away to rented properties. As I am on benefits, I can't afford good-quality flats, and I feel so angry as I should be in a top-level job, owning a good house, a car in the driveway, and have a secure private pension.

My past experiences help me, but sometimes I need help and don't know where to turn. Once I came round in the kitchen holding my hand under the cold tap as it was scalded. I have no idea what happened. Through all this, I received little help from the health service; they were just trying to work out suitable drugs. I always found my doctors very unhelpful; when I was first diagnosed, they didn't give me any advice or information about epilepsy. I used my experiences with my sister, studied the subject, and found that my "training" in the conflict was useful as I knew how to cope with emergencies. I wasn't frightened by it and managed to live as I used to, although other people's ignorance stopped me.

After the first few years, my doctors concluded that I was untreatable, unresponsive to drugs, and I began to feel that the appointments were only to check if I was still alive and try out a new drug to which I often had a bad reaction. One affected my vision so badly I was nearly blind. I kept asking my doctor to remove the drug, which he refused to do. After two years, he lost his temper and yelled at me to be blind or have fits—it was my choice. However, when I saw him again, the epilepsy nurse scheme [nurse-led epilepsy services] had been introduced, and he was very friendly. He agreed to take away the drug, but I found the nurse difficult to get on with and had little help from her.

At thirty-nine, I was sent to a specialist center in England for a review and had my first MRI. This showed that one side of my hippocampus (a part of the brain) was shrunken, but no reason was found. That result eventually led to the diagnosis of non-epileptic attack disorder. Otherwise, no results were found to help me. I had a vagus nerve stimulator implanted, but it only worsened my condition and was finally removed, though the metal wires were left in place, which stops me from having any more MRIs. I learned about post-traumatic stress disorder when I read about World War One and recognized some symptoms of shell shock in myself. It was confirmed when I saw a play about terrorism during which the theater used too-realistic sounds of bombs and gunshots. I was so badly affected that I couldn't leave the theatre for nearly an hour. I sought help for it and received counseling at a government-funded organization. It only worsened my condition as I had to relive the scenes of terror.

I'd been trying to find a cause for my epilepsy from the start and searched for information about the effects of post-traumatic stress disorder. There is little written about it in popular books for the general public, and I had to study research papers, etc. Finally, I found enough evidence that severe emotional trauma as a child releases stress chemicals that damage the developing brain, which I took to my doctor to ask for another review at the specialist center as there aren't sufficient resources where I live. They refused me, and I had to argue the case when I learned that a patient has the rights to be referred to another area in the UK if they can't be helped at home. I finally went to the center when I was sixty, and using modern diagnostic equipment, they found I was having seizures that didn't register on the EEG as well as ones that did. I saw a neuropsychiatrist who diagnosed dissociation and confirmed that my hippocampus may have been damaged during the trouble I had experienced. However, my own doctors have been unhelpful. I received the results in March, but my doctor wouldn't see me until June. He referred me to a neuropsychologist, but there is only one specialist in Northern Ireland, who has a long waiting list. Again, I'm learning about it through my own studies and groups found on Facebook.

90

Person Who Is Now Free of PNES, USA

I was diagnosed with psychogenic non-epileptic seizures in January 2014. It was at the end of a four-day hospital stay where I had every imaginable test that the doctors could think of to explain the violent convulsions I had, which so closely resembled grand mal seizures. I can still close my eyes and remember that day, my friend snickering as he heard the doctor tell me my diagnosis was psychogenic non-epileptic seizures, or PNES, because when saying "PNES," it really does sound like you're trying to say "penis." That has become a great icebreaker for many of my fellow PNES-ers, and it's important to find something to laugh about, so why not that.

Well, I was sent packing that day with instructions to find a stress-free environment (not helpful) and told the tragic news that there was no recovery possible, and no method of treatment except to lower stress in my life. This was perplexing at best. I felt like I was just handed a paper encoded with invisible ink and told that the decoder is somewhere with Bigfoot. I had not been given any real answers to get better, and I strongly felt that hospitals were where you go to find answers for the really scary and hard problems—well, it's not, not for us. They don't have the answers for most of us; as I learned over that next six months, the answers were within me.

I guess the first thing you should know about me is that I am extremely stubborn; the best way to get me to do something is to try and convince me that it's impossible. I just don't believe in that word, honestly. They said no recovery, and I was spending the majority of my day in or recovering from these episodes, which were pretty painful. I just wouldn't allow myself to believe it—just because the answer hadn't been found yet didn't mean there wasn't one. I was thirty-four years old, and I had two very young children—this was not how my life was going down. I was making deals with God and was going to learn as much as I could about my body and brain and fixing myself (as I didn't have doctors to help with this). The deal with

God was not to recover and never look back, but was about wanting to help others once He helped me sort out the broken pieces of my life.

Well, after six months of grueling and gut-wrenching self-work in deconstructing "Me," I was seizure-free and starting to help others discover how to do it for themselves. I had created a YouTube channel to document everything I learned throughout the process. I didn't have doctors to explain how it was possible, so I used simple language.

Then I came across neuroplasticity, and it all made sense how psychogenic non-epileptic seizures and other "mental disorders," which are all categorized as unresolvable, can be resolved after all. I searched medical journals to see which parts of the brains in patients with psychogenic non-epileptic seizures are atrophied or overused based on their size from scans, and that gave me a great head start into explaining it, and then coming up with exercises and practices for people to use.

Now I must say, it's not for wimps—recovery is about getting real honest with yourself about how you're living life. If psychogenic non-epileptic seizures is the cause, then there is a lot of healing to do, and you are the one in the control seat. (That was my case, so I know). I had to exit some people from my life, learn some new life skills, create some self-helping and coping social etiquette and form, and most of all, get out of the past and stay out. I had to forgive a lot; surprisingly, I owed myself a large share of forgiveness too. I share a lot in my YouTube video blog of recovery, and I must say that getting what I now refer to as a "huge red-flag disorder," psychogenic non-epileptic seizures is the best thing that happened to me. My eyes are opened, and I owe it all to love—love of my two friends who stayed with me for twenty-four-hour shifts for three months, love of the people who let me cry on their shoulders, love of the many people I had found through Facebook and YouTube, love of people who let me into their lives and share the healing power of companionship and support, and love of my Heavenly Father, who never left me alone through it all. Ironically, psychogenic non-epileptic seizures are so often caused from the antithesis of love, leaving the only antidote to be true love. Truly liking and loving yourself is the most potent formula for people with psychogenic non-epileptic seizures, and you can't do that with all the old versions of your past hanging around like a noose. Take hope; recovery is possible for you! And it's free.

91

Person with Epilepsy and PNES, USA

Seizures in themselves are frustrating. Epileptologists do not always read electroencephalograms in the same manner, or rather don't agree with the findings. I remember having issues as a child when I would get a strange feeling in my stomach. I didn't tell anyone as I didn't want restrictions. I remember the first time I lost consciousness coming out of the bath; I had to stay in bed the rest of the day. Other episodes occurred that were most likely syncope, but this was years ago and a neurologist was unheard of in my little country town.

Instances of lost consciousness occurred throughout my life. I have lived an "on the bus, off the bus" existence with regard to epilepsy versus psychogenic non-epileptic seizures. I had years of counseling, hoping that would stop the frequent spells of loss of consciousness. I was a research patient at a university using biofeedback in attempts to control my autonomic nervous system to avoid orthostatic hypotension—I was quite good at that, but events would still occur on rare occasions. I was still maintained on an anti-epileptic drug at that time. As a veteran, I was seen at a specialized hospital and sent home on an anti-epileptic drug. Two days later, someone else had reviewed the reading and called to tell me to stop the anti-epileptic drug. I had a neurologist that did frequent spinal taps; thank goodness he was very good at it. I was hospitalized at one time for an arteriogram but had pulmonary arrest during the procedure. I was put on so many medications at one time that my electroencephalogram reading became too slow, and I was rushed to a university hospital by ambulance during the night. I was placed in a long-term monitoring facility where we all walked around with electroencephalogram-wired helmets for monitoring. By this point, I had had it. I just wanted to be told I was okay and to live my life without medication.

Effect on the rest of the family—when my daughter was little, the rule was if momma had a seizure in public, she was to take my purse and sit on me until help arrived. My husband became so frustrated that I remember him once stepping over me like one would ignore a child having a tantrum. We talk about those instances now, and he described the feeling of impotence in not being able to stop what was happening to me. I am a lucky one as we are still married after forty-seven years.

I myself feel great sadness that my condition caused so many traumas to my family and I missed things during my lifetime. I know that my events were non-epileptic, at least most of them were. When a neurologist I currently work with agreed that some of my events were indeed conversion reactions—they stopped. I do still have rare events now determined to be temporal lobe seizures found on electroencephalogram, but the bizarre frequent events have stopped.

I often ask why this all began, and I have no answer. Since I work in neurology, I know that some form of sexual trauma often precipitates the events, but I had none. It did not provide me with positive attention, only embarrassment. Do I have a possible theory? Yes. I question if when I would get that "strange feeling" I would panic, which would lead to the events. I now know when I get that strange feeling to simply relax, and it will either pass or evolve into a seizure with a short period of altered awareness. They are not violent, and it is rare that I fall since I generally know when they are about to occur.

When I look back at those non-epileptic events, I in general would remember all that occurred, and although I might have been tired due to the physical or emotional strain, it was not the desperate need to sleep as I experience now. Having had non-epileptic spells, I will probably always search for the reason precipitating them and question why simply understanding and accepting the diagnosis stopped them. How I wish it had been explained to me years ago as I know I was not consciously causing them. I can forgive myself and move on.

92

Person with PNES, UK

I'm walking around this old German bunker, viewing these amazing art installations, and all I can think about is the excruciating pain I am feeling radiating through my body. My bones feel like they are breaking more and more with every step I take, the glorious repercussions of a car accident I had just a couple months earlier. My breaths are getting faster, my heart is thumping so hard, I feel like it's about to jump out of my chest; I feel sick, like really, really sick. I look around to find a seat, but they are all occupied. I'm feeling so dizzy, the pain is getting worse, my vision is going black, and I'm down. I wake up to find myself somewhere strange: I am on my own, in a foreign city, and I am in a hospital. That was my first experience of a non-epileptic attack.

With a CT scan of my brain, I am told I do not have epilepsy and am discharged the next day. I'm told to rest for the day. I've been sleeping for hours to wake up to someone pounding my chest and breathing into my mouth; my roommate thinks I've had a fit and stopped breathing. I'm shocked and scared, and a paramedic is now trying to take me back to hospital. What on earth is happening to me? What is wrong with me? Everything is moving so quickly. I'm meant to be flying home tomorrow, I don't want to be in the hospital, get me home, and I'm so scared! Three days of every scan under the sun and having a fit every afternoon, electrocardiogram, electroencephalogram, CT, magnetic resonance imaging, my brain is fine, my heart is fine, and nothing is changing. What on earth is going on with my body? I'm losing control of my body, I become tense, so tense I'm shivering. I feel so sick I want to gag, the room feels like it's spinning around and around, and my vision slowly blacks out as if the opacity of a black screen just gets darker and darker until I can no longer see. I crouch down and feel my surroundings with my hands to allow myself to lie down until I eventually erupt and the cycle begins again. It's now been three days, and this hospital is the most depressing place in the world. I can't stop crying, I don't know what is happening, is it serious, what could it be?

It's taking a toll. My tutor comes in during the day and tries to get my spirits up; an hour after he leaves, I'm back to the same miserable state. Finally, when I was about to be discharged, my doctor asks me one more time if there is anything I haven't mentioned. I inform him that I was recently diagnosed with post-traumatic stress disorder after being involved in a car accident. It was as if a light switched on in his head, but I was so desperate to go home after days of pure misery that he didn't say anything, but did ask me to see a psychologist about this at home.

Weeks go by, and the attacks don't stop. I've seen doctor after doctor, all of which want me to wait months for a neurologist. I have done so much research by this point, reading about sleep apnea, narcolepsy, postural tachycardia syndrome, but none of these can explain why I am having seizures if I don't have epilepsy. I speak to my cognitive behavioral therapist who is treating me for post-traumatic stress disorder; she is telling me that she thinks I am having disassociation episodes, what could be a conversion disorder. Back to the search engine I go. I'm researching as much as I can until I come along a condition called psychogenic non-epileptic seizures, and after much research, although my symptoms fit, it sounds a lot like they are calling these seizures fake. So I can't have that condition because what is happening to me is far from fake. Why on earth would someone fake such a horrific experience? It doesn't make any sense. Nope—definitely not my condition.

A couple weeks later, I get my full discharge note. It's all in German, so I cannot understand anything, except for one thing that is almost a replica of a condition I have read about. I quickly translated it: "Having reviewed her scans and electro-encephalogram and upon confirmation of her suffering post-traumatic stress disorder, I can confirm that the patient is suffering with psychogenic non-epileptic seizures, and she should seek treatment from an appropriate psychologist." My world collapsed, this can't be it, they feel too real, they are saying that I am faking this, why would I fake this, it's bringing me nothing but misery, it is affecting my work, my education, my ability to go outside. Why on earth would I bring this upon myself? NO. He is wrong. There is something seriously wrong with me, and no one is doing anything to help. Why doesn't anyone understand that I am losing control of my own body? This is not normal, nor is it okay.

I take this note to my therapist and explain what it says. I tell her that it must be wrong, but then she went away and discussed it with some of her colleagues. A week later, she tells me she agrees with the diagnosis. REALLY? So you think I'm faking too? I just wanted to curl up into a ball and cry until I had no tears left. She was speaking to me and explaining how it is basically the same as disassociation and that she knows it is not fake, but as she was speaking, I was dazing and began to feel it again, my body tensing, the feeling of sick clogging up my throat, the black screen getting darker and darker, the dizziness. I wake up to her dabbing me with cold wet tissues. My eyes are struggling to adjust to the brightness in the room, my head is pounding, and I feel like my body is so heavy I can barely lift a finger. Her voice is really distant. So distant that it is inaudible. I just want to sleep. It takes me about ten minutes before I can hear her voice properly, before I can possibly sit up again.

This is so embarrassing, someone is watching me lose control of my body, and it's painstaking to know that I'm out cold with no idea of what is happening around me. Now I'm up, I still don't feel okay yet, still a bit dizzy and nauseous, but my therapist is so intent that I must be fine ten minutes later and it's time to leave. Feeling embarrassed, I get up to leave. As I head to the elevator, everything is spinning, I need to sit, but not here, and I try to go a little farther. I see the bright, colored blobs that could only be the seats in reception I vaguely remember, so I walk toward a blob and sit, dropping my head between my legs, and all I remember is waking to the yelling of a lady shouting "Crash team!" Wonderful.

I often wake up and ask the person who looked after me what they saw, what did they say, what was their reaction? Were they traumatized? Sometimes I'm given a weird look, as if asking why do I want to know. I want to know because while I may be used to it, and you may be used to it, I am so very aware that other people are not. I still remember the first time I saw someone else have a seizure; it scared me. A lot. They looked so defenseless and strange. I now must look the same to others. I remember when my friends at university first saw their first bad seizure while we were on a study trip. There were tears. I hated scaring them. They're used to it now, but it's so embarrassing and leaves me feeling so vulnerable and awkward. You wake up to the room staring back at you, and it's so awkward. People have this odd, sympathetic smile that just makes you want the world to swallow you up from how horrible you feel. That's all on top of the fact that you feel like you have just gone ten rounds in a kick-boxing match, and the idea of even lifting a finger at the time feels as if you're about to lift eighty-kilogram weights. What people don't tend to understand is that the fear is not only of having a seizure, but of what happens to you while you're out cold. I'm probably on the floor, my body uncontrollably jerking with no control over what people do to me. Some people try to hold me down, usually leaving me with painful bruises from their tight grip. Some people have put my head on their knees and really strained my already-injured neck muscles, and it felt like I had torn something for a while. And some people just hold me in such weird ways that caused me to dislocate my shoulder. Twice. It's not just what people that are caring for you do, though; sometimes you may be somewhere strange—for example a train station. You may be alone, and you do not know what types of people are around. I know of a woman who had a seizure while alone at a train station and woke up with her trousers by her ankles. I don't think I need to explain this any further. This by far is my biggest fear. Not only do you lose control, other people can gain it. I'm lucky that I get a warning; I can try and make sure I'm safe. But more needs to be done to give people with conditions like these some security.

My life after diagnosis? Well, it's not peachy. It's been a tough road; after months of denial and hope of another answer, I've had to admit to myself that these seizures are psychogenic and accept that maybe a different form of treatment is something that will help. My life is so different now. I have so many restrictions, studying has gotten so much harder, I cannot go past one assignment without a deadline extension, during assessment periods the seizures get so much worse, and work had become increasingly hard to juggle. I was one of the top diamond and watch advisors in my store for so long, but after the seizures, everything changed. My sales dropped drastically. I didn't have the energy, and I was always cautious of straining my body so that I didn't have a seizure. If I did have a seizure, then I would be out back for a couple hours, and then beg to not be sent home as I was so scared of it causing me to lose my job. My colleagues were really great about everything, especially my manager. Whenever it would happen, my colleagues would just be so great with making sure they don't do anything that I've informed the manager I don't want anyone to do. Just leave me to it. I'll be fine. I don't want any attention please! I do get a warning, so I will make sure I am safe before I pass out. After a while I felt like I needed a fresh start and felt my manager was getting frustrated with the difference in me, and so I decided it was time to move on. New job and a few months in, they were also brilliant. My previous job accomplishments helped me get the job easily; they didn't even think about my condition. In the times I did have seizures there, they were so good to me, and it was so comforting to see that although previously I was very worried they would get rid of me, they didn't when they saw it while I was still on probation. However, a few months later, I realized I just couldn't juggle my condition with work and university, so I had to make a choice, and of course I chose university. It's not made life easy. I'm strained for money, and I miss the social break from coursework that my job gave me, but I couldn't juggle it all anymore. It was proving impossible to do both, and my education is everything to me.

Paramedics? Terrible. They are all bubbly and friendly until they hear the term *non-epileptic seizures*. The first thing they say is say, "Oh, so you're having pseudoseizures." NO. They are not "pseudo." They are so real. The expression on the faces of the paramedics after are just different, and they treat you as if you are a time waster. I didn't ask for you to be here! Ninety percent of the time, an ambulance is never called because I am so clear in begging everyone around me not to call an ambulance if I have a seizure. I told my colleagues at work and peers at university within the first few days of meeting them about my condition, even though I didn't have to, just so I could make sure that they don't call an ambulance if it happens. I hate the way the paramedics make me feel. I remember once I was starting to wake up from a seizure, and the paramedic had pricked my finger a few moments after I started to feel in the room again. I was still very hazy and in my own world; I jerked when she pricked me because of the strong sensation, at a time when sensations were only just returning to me. She was horrible to me from them on, and I heard her talking to someone and referring to my seizure as "whatever it was that she just did." It was like a punch to the stomach. I felt so humiliated; my heart completely sank into a pit of self-hatred. Paramedics really need to be more aware of this condition. It was hard enough to accept that this is what's wrong with me, so when people like her treat me in that way because of it, it just makes it so much harder. It sends me back into denial. She's rude to me because she believes I am doing this to myself. WHY WOULD I PUT MYSELF THROUGH SUCH HUMILIATION?! She was just shouting at me to speak straight away. "Come on. tell us your name already, we can't do anything if you don't talk, come on - we need to get you up now, tell us your name!" I cannot explain what it is like to wake up from a seizure to this. She truly believed I was faking and just refusing to speak. I wanted so much to just shout at her to be quiet; I didn't have the energy to even open my mouth. I wanted to burst out into tears, and I did shed a few. Why me, why? Can someone please just hand me a different diagnosis and tell me it will be okay? That was all I wanted, but sadly, I know that is not going to happen. So I just have to live with it, but that doesn't make it any easier when these things happen.

Treatments? Here's the worst bit, under the National Health Service I have suffered with this condition for two years with absolutely no treatment offered to me. The most I received was a prescription to raise my blood pressure. From the way I have been treated by paramedics and doctors after hearing about my condition, I have been left feeling too ashamed to go back and persist that I need help. I find medical practitioners very intimidating and struggle to speak to them. My previous treatment of cognitive behavioral therapy was for post-traumatic stress disorder, but when my therapist learned of the psychogenic non-epileptic seizures, she attempted to treat me for it, too. The treatment didn't help any of my conditions, and I was referred for further long-term support, which I never received. My solicitor has finally put funding forward for me to start some eye movement desensitization and reprocessing treatment, as he feels I desperately need it. I have had four sessions so far. To be honest, I'm not finding it helpful at all yet, but I continue to keep an open mind as I feel like it is now my only hope for possibly getting better. Is it fair that there is so little that can be done for people with my condition? It is a very common illness, yet in two years, I haven't come across one practitioner that is aware of it.

Family? Well, that's another struggle. I don't come from the typical clued-up and super-caring family. I come from an Arab family, and we're all very awkward when it comes to emotion. My sister is so avoidant of speaking about my seizures, my brother just freaks out if I have a seizure near him and will never speak about it to me, and my mother—well, she's pretty clueless when it happens, she doesn't know what to do and just gets super-awkward. My dad is the worst of them. The first time he saw me have a seizure, he decided to grab me by the leg and try to shake me out if it. I cannot describe how horrified I was when I woke up. So completely shocking and embarrassing. Even though they are the closest people to me, my family members have seen only a few seizures. The only time they will see one is when I have no place or time to hide. All I do is hide at home if I don't feel well. Get into bed and turn the lights off to make out as if I just went to sleep so that no one comes in. They think I very rarely have any seizures, but really, I have so many while hiding under my duvet just so I can avoid the sheer awkwardness and embarrassment that they make me feel.

Non-epileptic seizures completely turned my life around. I speak mostly of the difficulties I have faced, but what I will say is that it has made me a much stronger person. It's not easy. You have your up and down days, your empowered days, and your seriously depressed days. The quality of life with this condition is very poor, with really underdeveloped treatment, but it doesn't mean you have to let it beat you. As hard as it is, I will never let it beat my goal of finishing university with my friends. Although it has reduced the amount I go out, when I do I try to really enjoy myself. I try to live as normal a life as I can. You gain a view of the world that many people don't have; it shows you how quickly things can change and how much you need to live your life as hard as it may be. I feel like if my post-traumatic stress disorder eventually is successfully treated, it will break so many more barriers for me, and my life will probably get even better. But until then, I will always try to keep positive because I know every day I am surviving and that is something not a lot of people understand.

I do feel like I would probably be in a much better position if I had practitioners around me that understood my condition. Other than in Germany, not one doctor I have come across already knew of psychogenic non-epileptic seizures; most of them don't take the time to find out for you. I have absolutely no support network other than my solicitor and now my eye movement desensitization and reprocessing therapist, who don't even understand psychogenic non-epileptic seizures themselves but are trying to get to know it or piece it together with me. They are the only people who assure me that I am not crazy. It would make the world of difference to have doctors around me that would reassure me. I'm at the point where I feel guilty if any medical practitioner comes across a seizure as I feel like I am wasting their time. This is not right. I am a human being who is suffering from a very real condition, and it took me two years to finally realize it. I hope this book will finally spread awareness that is desperately needed.

93

Person with PNES, USA

I am eighteen years old. I suffer with what has been diagnosed as "pseudoseizures." These seizures began when I was only thirteen years old. I was attending a normal school. I had many friends, a loving family, and a very supportive boyfriend. I was on my school wrestling team, I made great grades, and I loved my life. I was very happy. I noticed that some mornings when I would wake up, I would have bruises or scratches on my body that were not there when I had gone to sleep. Sometimes I would wake up in the shower with shampoo still in my hair. I had no idea what to think, and I can't explain why, but I was afraid to tell my mother about experiencing these strange things. But when it got worse, I had to.

My mother took me to the doctor, and we were referred to a neurologist. The day of that appointment is the first day I heard the word *seizure*. After talking to multiple professionals in the medical field, it was determined that I could no longer be on any sports team because it was too dangerous. I continued to support my wrestling teammates, who were like family to me. I traveled with the team to see them compete at the state competition. That was when I had a seizure in front of people for the first time. My mother's best friend was there, her son wrestled, so she stayed with me until it was over.

My mother decided to take me back to another neurologist. It was decided I needed medicine. Over the course of these five years, I have been on multiple medications. After nothing seemed to work, and years went by, my mother took me to see a Lyme disease specialist. It was determined I did not have Lyme disease. After that, we traveled out of state to see an integrative medicine doctor. This doctor put me on a diet where I was not allowed any foods that contained dye, and I was not allowed any food that contained gluten. I was miserable. He also gave me multiple pills to consume every day. My seizures got worse and worse, and I decided to end this process.

Eventually I was taken to have an electroencephalogram, where they monitored me for a few days through a camera. After the third day, using sleep deprivation, I had my seizure. Doctors concluded I had no abnormal brain activity, and it was determined that I had pseudoseizures. After this, I was to see a psychiatrist and psychologist, who I formed a relationship with. It could not be determined why I had these seizures. They told me that usually these seizures are caused by a traumatic event in someone's life. But I've spent years trying to figure out what that event is, and I can't. Together, they prescribed me different medications, but none of them could fix me. Being a teenage girl and going through this was very depressing. At one point, I was on so many different medications that I became suicidal. I attempted to end my own life. The life that I had loved until these "things" began.

With my family's support, I stopped taking all of the medication, stopped seeing my doctors, and just took one day at a time. When I would have a seizure, I would take a nap, take two painkillers, and continue with life. When I have my seizures, I go blank. I pass out, unconscious. I then begin convulsing, crying, screaming, jerking, and twitching. I do not bite my tongue; I do not void my bowels. I have viewed video footage of one of my seizures, and they are terrifying. They look like an actual seizure. When I wake up, I am unaware of what has happened. I also lose memory of the full day I experienced before having my seizure. I rarely recover my memory of how my day went before the seizure. It is truly upsetting.

My seizures got so bad that I stopped going to school and did something called "home hospital." This is a form of home schooling where a teacher would come to my house to work with me. I had to stop going to my public school because I had so many seizures at school and I was bullied for it.

My fiancé and I have now been together for six years. When I was only fifteen years old, I got pregnant with our daughter. I was so terrified. I couldn't help but worry about having a seizure and hurting her and myself. In order to have a healthy pregnancy, I decided to stop taking my anti-epileptic medication, which was the only medicine I was on for my seizures at that time. I don't know how, or why. I cannot explain it, my doctors cannot explain it, but my seizures almost completely stopped. I only had three seizures the entire pregnancy. For nine months and four days, I only had three seizures. For my fiancé, my family, and myself, it was a complete mystery and shock.

My daughter is my absolute world. After I gave birth to her, I decided to attend a school that allowed me to bring my daughter to school with me every day. She stays in day care while I go to the other side of the building and go to school. It is the best decision I have ever made. I'm proud to say I graduate this May. My daughter is now two. I went an extremely long time without having seizures. I stopped having them when I was halfway through my pregnancy. I went almost two years without having one. But recently, they have unfortunately started again. I have an amazing support system, and I am never left alone. My school has a clinic full of nurses who love me and support me. When I have a seizure, they take care of me.

I have decided not to seek medical help for my seizures. The heartbreak of hearing a medical professional tell you that you are unfixable creates a feeling in your heart that makes you feel broken. I have worked on myself as a person and done everything in my power to keep my seizures under control. They have been very bad for the past three months, but I have recently met a woman who helped me to find God. Forming a close relationship with Christ has helped me very much. Also, doing activities that I enjoy, such as art projects, helps too. Through church, my mentor, my amazing daughter and fiancé, my father, my family, and my selfless and perfect mother, who is my biggest supporter, I am able to live a life that I love. I recently got accepted into college, where I will get my doctorate in physical therapy. I am trying to just live.

There is a part of me that would love to know exactly why I have these seizures. There is a part of me that wishes I was fixable. But when I really think about it, I am a very lucky person. Pseudoseizures are a horrible thing to live with, but life is manageable. If you are determined enough, it is possible to have a happy life.

94

Person with Epilepsy and PNES, USA

I am a sixty-five-year-old Caucasian female. I was born and raised in the United States with good health care all my life. I am a college graduate, and I've traveled extensively and lived in Italy for two years of my adult life. My overall health is generally good except for my seizure disorder brought on by two consecutive car accidents when I was thirteen years old. I had my first seizure at that time, in 1965. Emergency Room people dismissed it as stress and my menstrual cycle. I was diagnosed with grand mal seizures when my second seizure took place in 1970 at the age of eighteen.

Electroencephalograms over the years confirmed, and I continued to have, grand mal seizures until about 1989. I blacked out during these seizures and only remember dreaming. When I came to consciousness, I was washed out and needed sleep. I then had no seizures until about 1999. That's when my episodes changed in nature to the non-epileptic type. I remember these episodes until Emergency Room people give me medication to relax me.

For my epileptic seizures, I was given an anti-epileptic drug, which increased in dosage over the years. After taking that for fifty years, I began to show signs of osteoporosis in my left hip. I was sent to a doctor who then changed my medication. I continued to have non-epileptic episodes, two to four times a year.

Usually my non-epileptic episodes wake me in the night with nausea and body shaking. My body feels like electricity shooting through me and would make different parts shake uncontrollably. I begin to rock back and forth, sometimes drawing my legs up to my torso. My face is contorted, and my speech is slurred. I cannot respond verbally; however, my hearing is acute. My walk is contorted, if I can walk at all. I am semi-conscious. Sometimes my torso would raise up off the bed. On one occasion, I verbally squealed. My episodes come in waves of shaking, usually three per episode, with several minutes in between of relaxed muscles and completely washed out feelings. Viruses, emotional pain, and dehydration have all been said to bring on these episodes. I am totally unable to keep hydrated. I cannot take enough water to keep me from getting sick. I started drinking sports drinks to try and maintain my hydration level. I limit my outside time and activity due to dehydration. By the time I felt parched, it usually was too late to take in enough liquid. I am very sensitive to hot and cold weather.

I have been under a doctor's care since 1970. Due to insurance restrictions, most of the time I had neurological care. Over the years, I had been tested many times, always confirming the grand mal epileptic seizure disorder. Most doctors just gave me an anti-epileptic drug because it seemed to control my seizures. Due to resumed seizure activity, I was sent to another doctor in late 2012. In 2016, I saw yet another doctor. He tested me and changed my medication. I had never heard of a non-epileptic episode, but he told me my episodes were caused by a deep psychological reason, one I may not even be aware of.

When it comes to emergency medical technicians, I appreciate their care. However, *they need much more training in epileptic disorders!* I have had many emergency medical technicians tell me I was *not* having a seizure! This only makes me feel worse! Many have tried to get me to talk to them. I cannot when I am shaking, and can only speak slurred and slow when I am not shaking! Many try to put thermometers in my mouth!! I've never tried to swallow my tongue, but I am incapable of holding a thermometer in my mouth due to the uncontrolled movement. Emergency vehicles have bright lights, especially at night. This just blinds me! My hearing is acute, so I hear all the laughter, jokes, and diagnoses! I need to hear that I am in a safe place getting the help I need.

When it comes to Emergency Room personnel, usually these people are keenly qualified. However, nurses try to put thermometers in my mouth. If I don't respond, they usually try to speak louder, not understanding that I can't respond. I wear a Medical Alert necklace, but not one medical person has ever checked it.

My mother always got me the care I needed. My husband of forty-five years had always gotten me the care I needed. No one has ridiculed me for having this sickness. My husband has spent many sleepless nights in the Emergency Room, and I am so blessed to have him! He is a godsend. Due to this condition, we agreed not to have children. I am blessed to have many loving relatives and have not felt deprived. I have always taken my medications faithfully, so I can drive, attend school, and work. I need more sleep than most, but that was not a problem in my life. I feel I lead a normal life.

My concerns are that I am no longer on anti-epileptic medication. The doctor hasn't completely convinced me I am no longer epileptic. I had not had an episode of any kind since starting an anti-depressant in mid-2017. I feel better all around. I tried not to let epilepsy rule my life. However, it was always in the background. I no longer have that worry. This feeling is still new to me, and I wonder when I no longer became epileptic.

The doctor suggested I see a psychologist and that treatment could be difficult and last as long as twenty years. At this time, I have opted not to take that course. At sixty-five years old, I don't see the advantage. I am a very spiritual person and believe God knows all. I have put it in HIS hands. I am grateful for the medication that has relieved my non-epileptic episodes. I now live a normal life!

I am thrilled to have this opportunity to share my experiences. If it can help anyone else in the world live a better life, I am happy to be a part of that.

95

Partner of Person with Epilepsy and PNES, USA

My wife and I have been married for over forty-five years. As long as I have known her, she has remained active. She is intelligent, articulate, and the most thoughtful and caring person I've ever met. The last year or so, after a medicine change, she has renewed energy, emotional strength, and a positive outlook. The information provided here is given to help others who encounter similar circumstances.

I was twenty-two years old when we married. At the time, I didn't fully comprehend all of the aspects of my future bride's condition. However, I didn't perceive it as a reason not to get married. The first time she had a seizure, I was a bit unnerved, mainly because I had never seen anyone have a seizure and I simply didn't know what to do. We had gone to see a movie, and during one disturbing scene, she had to leave. I followed her out, and she collapsed in the lobby and exhibited the symptoms with which I would later become familiar—semi-consciousness, stiff body, facial twitches, and uncontrollable crying. I was afraid for her, but later came to understand what was happening and my role during these episodes. Over the first three decades of our relationship, she had a couple of seizures, usually brought on by severe emotional distress (such as a death in the family) or sickness. During those times, we would make a trip to the Emergency Room, and I would turn the treatment over to qualified medical personnel.

During the last five years or so, her seizures became more frequent. There were two factors, I believe. First, because of osteoporosis concerns, her medication was changed. I don't believe the new medication worked as well—later believing (from conversations with doctors) that it was probably the wrong treatment at the time. Second, there was the increased stress of growing older—more sickness and emotional stress, deaths in the family, etc.

I learned that major triggers of my wife's episodes during this time were emotional stress and dehydration—brought on by sickness or environmental conditions. At times, she could be strong emotionally, such as withstanding bad news about a relative. When my father passed away in 2013, she stood firmly by me. However, when her aunt passed away, she had an episode in her hospital room. I believe she was as close to my dad as she was her aunt, so the difference in response is unknown, possibly fatigue.

For this writing, I'll classify environmental conditions in two ways, physical and spiritual. Home environment: we have multiple humidifiers within the home to help maintain the correct humidity levels (to help with dehydration). Top-grade air purifier/filters are placed in strategic areas to keep the air as fresh as possible—no very strong scents allowed. We do have scented candles, etc., but they are few and very subtle. She loves plants, and we have some in the house, but again, those with allergic potential are either kept outside or not at all. Spiritual: we do our best to make our home as peaceful as possible. Let me say this, we are devout, active Christians. We believe the presence of God and His Spirit in our lives and in our home to be the MAIN contributing factor in the love and peace that exists here. We NEVER fight or quarrel. We compliment one another and express our love for each other often. We NEVER leave without a loving goodbye. We recognize God's blessing and will not take the idea of HIS divine influence lightly.

During the last five years or so, my wife would have several episodes a year, requiring a trip to the Emergency Room. I had learned to recognize when an episode was imminent. She would struggle to maintain her composure. She would be on the verge of crying or exhibit signs of duodenal distress, holding her stomach as if she had a stomach ache. Most often, she would complain of nausea. I could tell she was dehydrated—skin dry and lips parched. She would possibly begin to rock back and forth, front to back. She didn't lose consciousness and would resist my insistence on taking her to the Emergency Room. After about half an hour of these symptoms, I would insist that we go to the Emergency Room; only then would she capitulate. Often, while we were in the car, she would experience increased symptoms—crying uncontrollably, facial twitches, and bodily tics. At the hospital, during the "deepest' cycles, she would not allow me to touch her. She could communicate, but only between the evidence of symptoms; they would come in waves, seemingly worse each time.

In the Emergency Room, because of my experience, I would actually prescribe her treatment to the Emergency Room personnel. I worked with the doctors and nurses to provide fluids because she was almost dehydrated, as well as medication for nausea and to help her rest. The doctors always followed my instructions. Once the treatment began, the symptoms would subside, and she would fall asleep. I was grateful for that. After several hours, she would awaken and we would go home for her to rest. She would be exhausted from the ordeal; it would take a couple of days to fully recover.

Mid-year 2016, during our visit to the doctor, he asked me to video one of my wife's episodes (if she had one) and allow him to see it. In August, she became ill and had an episode that required a visit to the Emergency Room. We followed the procedures I outlined above and videoed it. It was one of the most painful things I've ever had to endure. My wife was suffering, and I'm holding into an electronic device instead of her hand. During the episodes, although I knew what was happening, it was terribly painful to watch someone you love so dearly have to endure it. During our lives, I learned to temper the input to my wife's world. I would try to tell her disappointing news at specific tines, insist on a drink to increase hydration or work with her on which foods to eat. When we traveled, I would make sure we did so in stages so she wouldn't get too tired. Environmental conditions, including in the car, were (and are) at her command—her comfort was (and is) paramount over mine; I can adjust easier.

April 2017, and with the prescription of an anti-depressant by the doctor, everything has changed. My wife no longer takes anti-epileptic medication. As she says, "The doctor gave me my life back." She is teaching again, taking yoga, she has more energy, sleeps more soundly, has a positive outlook, and can withstand the triggers that formerly gave her trouble. The fact that we can write about these things is a testament to how much has changed.

We are thankful to God for His blessing and for allowing us to be partnered with the doctor. For those who have a loved one who suffers with these symptoms, learn the triggers that affect them and the treatment that works. Best of all, find someone who can review the symptoms and prescribe an effective treatment.

96

Person with PNES, USA

Writing this is in itself therapeutic. And to review my experience with the possibility of helping others opens an entirely new vista. Being a practicing psychologist for over thirty years, I have seen the presence of non-epileptic seizures increase within my own clientele. The root cause has always been some sort of trauma, and the seizure itself is an intense panic attack. Survivors of abuse, war, prolonged or intense grief, and physical pain can manifest this symptom, as well as those exposed to personally terrifying or shocking occurrences. In addition, persons in a relationship with this individual, including family and intimate relationships, friends, colleagues, and treatment personnel, are affected. The circle of those involved can be extensive. It is time for this condition to be better understood and for sources of healing to become more effective; misdiagnosis prolongs and actually prevents the very healing we seek.

It was my doctor who first introduced me to the possibility of having non-epileptic seizures. Being quite certain that epilepsy was an inappropriate diagnosis for me, yet one given and sustained for years by respected, caring physicians, I sought his evaluation. Though the prescribed medications were effective to a degree, this diagnosis overlooked the true source of my dysfunction, the mental and emotional wounds. And until they were recognized, I could not be appropriately treated, and full healing would be impossible.

The diagnosis of epilepsy that I was inaccurately given was extremely frightening. To me, it indicated the occurrence of unpredictable episodes of falling out of consciousness and manifesting bizarre physical movements with no sense of control. The condition frightens most people who may, to defend against anxiety, view the patient with condescension and rejection. The factors of fear and isolation dramatically increase an individual's task of coping with the seizure itself, making a misdiagnosis quite disconcerting.

Though not certain when I was first considered epileptic, my first seizure occurred in May 1980 (four months before my thirtieth birthday), just moments before my initial hook-up to a dialysis machine and several days prior to receiving a kidney transplant from my sister. The thought of my blood being pulled from my body into a machine was terrifying, not simply because it was being removed from my body, but also because my body could no longer perform this vital function, which meant I could not manage my own existence and was totally dependent on others. Being in critical care and near death, the seizure, triggered from an unconscious level, prompted emergency medical measures. It was intense. I remained unconscious long enough for the hook up to be completed. I believe the seizure severed the purpose of removing my consciousness during this other, unbearable event. It was supremely effective.

I did not have another seizure for about twelve years but did experience periods of panic and deep fear. After two years of health probation, I pursued my doctorate in psychology and was required to undergo an intensive period of personal psychotherapy. It was this process that first opened my awareness to the unseen landscape of my childhood psyche, the intense, prolonged, and exceedingly hurtful relations and emotions of my life.

I had been told that at eighteen months of age, I underwent some sort of physical malfunction that provoked lifelong physical challenges. There has never been a certain diagnosis, but the left side of my body was temporarily paralyzed and my parathyroid glands became overactive. It was determined to be a sort of palsy.

The experience and its resulting dysfunction were extremely difficult for my family, but especially for me. Though physical attributes were tolerable, I developed a fragile self-concept and serious emotional wounds. Thus, in spite of having very significant advantages, I was hugely ill-equipped for life beyond high school, for college and adulthood. So upon reaching these years, emotional situations I encountered and created sometimes become overwhelming, with one even being life-threatening. Only as I learned about the unconscious level of my being, perceived its construction, and developed skills for healing barriers and entanglements was my psyche in its malformed condition capable of knowing and representing itself accurately, of forming healthy intimate relationships and seeing the world in any perspective other than as a victim. I had lived largely in survival mode and used the tool of repression to hide this reality. It was at thirty-two years old, when treated by doctors of psychology who were as qualified in their domain as my medical doctors were in theirs, that this depth of recovery began.

Despite, or maybe because of, the level of attention to my inner life, I had another seizure seven years later, soon after receiving my doctorate and not long after marrying. It happened as I first gained a sense that I had left my childhood home forever. My husband was not threatening, but fulfilling the task of separation/individuation from family and becoming a forever-responsible adult certainly was. My parents had supported me throughout life, and additionally, unhealed emotional wounds bonded us. Though well-acquainted with our unseen dynamics, having both re-experienced and expressed significant aspects in therapy, I was not fully healed. Nevertheless, over the next twelve years seizures occurred only several times, when I felt major threats. It was after separating from my husband and returning to my hometown that they increased and began to appear more often, primarily following perturbing family affairs, and often during sleep.

My new life focused on establishing a quality professional practice and healthy personal life. After five years I remarried, to a man who is himself a psychotherapist, and began avidly seeking alternative treatments for seizures along with following the medical ones. But as my security increased, seizures increased. This was puzzling, having thought emotional traumas were largely healed. However, I was learning from alternative sources, such as cranial-sacral therapy, reiki, and yoga, that the energy of trauma exists not just in mental and emotional realms but in our body itself, often until we feel safe or it is somehow deemed relevant by our unconscious. This fact, along with seeing that within my family a provocative level of tension could still arise to trigger the explosive reactions within, caused me to believe in a deeper or different diagnosis for the dysfunction.

My traditional physicians of internal medicine, psychiatry, and nephrology could not adequately explain these events to me or conceive of a disorder other than epilepsy. So it was at this point that I contacted the head of neurology at a hospital. On my first visit with the doctor, he said, "You have post-traumatic stress disorder with intense panic attacks in the form of seizures."

I believe that was in 2016. I was thrilled, for finally my emotional trauma was identified by the profession my family not only recognized but was hesitant to deny. Legitimacy of my emotional wounds spurred further healing within our family. Our transformation is a great joy. It was amazing to see how, with this accurate diagnosis, the stigma of me being epileptic simply fell away, revealing truths of family function that had to be faced, understood, and healed. I am fortunate to have a family capable of this task, for until the truths were brought forth, our past was a burden for each of us in our own way.

Seizures continue for me after times of significant stress. I am learning when this is. My degree is part of a holistic practice and has enabled innovative progress in this area. I am also extremely grateful for all the care I have and continue to receive.

97

Person with Epilepsy and PNES, USA

I am fifty-one years old. I have had seizures since I was seventeen. It started with grand mal seizures. Then, as I got into my late thirties, my doctor at that time also discovered that I had petit mal and stress seizures. However, he didn't call them that. He said I was faking it! I knew I wasn't faking it; I was fully aware that there was something else going on. However, I kept on seeing him for some reason. About a month later, I was bedridden for three months. I was having ten to twelve grand mal seizures a day. If it wasn't for my boyfriend (my husband now), I don't know what I would have done. There were many times he would have to carry me to the bathroom. He would bathe me, made all my meals, and still kept up his full-time job. He is, and always will be, my rock.

I remember my first stress seizure like it was yesterday. It was when I was still bedridden. My husband was helping me back to bed, and all of a sudden, I fell down like a rock. I was wide awake and having a grand mal seizure. I could feel everything. The pain was unbearable. I tried to talk, scream, make any kind of eye contact that I could to let my husband know that I was "awake" and can feel this, please help me. And I remember seeing my husband looking around not knowing what to do. I think he was scared just like me. Only in a different way. I recall him saying, "I love you; it's going to be okay." The seizure lasted for only about a minute and a half. For me, though, it felt so much longer. When it finally stopped, I remember just crying. Not knowing what just happened to me. I had never had any kind of stress seizures like that before.

So the stress seizures, which were aggressive, started happening a lot more often. I kept trying different doctors. A few said, "Stop stressing out." Well, I just didn't know what to do with that considering I used to stress out over everything: family, friends, household chores, not being able to pull my own weight around our home. I'll let you into a little secret—all of that was not anything to worry about at all.

Then I had the privilege of meeting my current doctor. When I met him, I was a wreck, so many seizures. At that point and time in my life, I didn't know how much this man would change my life. Because by this time, I had just accepted the fact that I had epilepsy. Nothing I could do about it. The stress seizures were still a big problem, but I tried to have a positive attitude about life in general. I have been seeing this doctor now for about six years. He has helped me in more ways than I could have ever imagined.

He tried increasing or decreasing doses of medicine. Slowly, but surely, I was having only four or five seizures a month, including the stress seizures. He was still not happy with having four or five seizures a month, though, and he wanted me to stop with the stress seizures. So he lowered the dose of one of my medicines, and after a few weeks, I went eight months free of stress seizures.

The things that my body has gone through over just the past nine years are unbelievable. I have rolled around in broken glass after dropping and then having a seizure way too many times. Hit my head so much and so hard that I have lost my memory of my husband, kids, parents, and myself; now that is scary. My daughter was visiting me one summer when I had a seizure, went to lie down, and then she heard me scream. I didn't know her, where I was, or myself. She was so afraid, my daughter called my husband. They took me to the hospital, where I stayed for about a week. One day I woke up, saw my beautiful girl, and said, "Where are we?" She cried and hugged me like never before. I have had countless black eyes, fat lips, and stiches in my head. You get the picture.

All of this time, I was determined that I was going to get better. To be "normal," whatever that is. It's not just up to the doctors and medicines. Don't get me wrong, they play the primary part in all of this, and we really have to listen to what they say. Yes, stress seizures are brought on by stress; however, that is life. Life is stressful. It's all about how we deal with it, that we can help ourselves to hopefully stop the stress seizures. I have learned that not everyone's problem is mine. They can actually handle it on their own. That's family, friends, and whoever it may be. There are times when we need to put ourselves first. And when it comes to your well-being, you have to come first. You're worth it.

I want to thank my husband, who is always there for me. You cleaned up more messes than you should have had to, my love. To my children for the times that I couldn't be there but you always understood, even though I know you still worry. To my mama, thank you for never underestimating me, and to my daddy in heaven, thank you for installing the positive attitude in me and the willpower to never give up.

98

Partner of Person with Epilepsy and PNES, USA

When I started seeing my wife in 2005, she was prone to violent shaking that was referred to as a "spell" by her neurologist at the time. As I had no idea what was going on, I started observing her habits. Soon, I came to realize that different forms of excitement could trigger her condition. One episode was while we were having sex. It was a total surprise! Getting too hot in the summertime was another cause. If she would get angry or afraid, zoom, there she goes. At first, they looked like normal grand mal seizures. As time went on, thought, she would start opening her eyes during these episodes and mention that she was feeling these things and not forgetting everything as she had in the past. This was the first indication I had that there was something different going on. Then, with the EEG studies, they would say that the "spells" were not epileptic.

My wife had a long history of medicine that she had tried over the years. She would get resistant to the medications that were being given to her at the time as well. She would go from one episode every week to as many as ten to twelve in a few months. Very fast decline in response to the treatment, and her neurologist would change her dose slightly, then wait until we came back again and do very little. This went on for a few years. I could not take all of the damage that she was doing to herself. She was constantly kicking her own butt by bouncing off things or breaking them. We were both feeling miserable. For a change of pace, we went for a walk in the woods for a scenic hike; next thing you know, I had to carry her out of the National Park over my shoulder uphill a quarter of a mile through the woods. I had to get her through the snow to the vehicle so that she didn't freeze to death. Again, an uphill battle to get her to safety. Sometimes walking through the parking lot, she stiffened up. I carried her like a board back to the vehicle and made sure she was okay.

Once, when her neurologist was gone, she had banged her head off the toilet and probably had a concussion. The neurologist on call gave her an intravenous medicine at a high dose, and she totally lost her memory. She didn't know her own name or that of her parents or children. I was the only name she could remember. The neurologist checked her for everything. He went so far as to do a spinal tap. He then said that she had herpes in her eye! This went on for over two weeks with no resolution in the hospital. She was finally released as an apparent invalid. Once the medicine wore off, she started remembering things quickly; in a few hours, she was back to normal. After that, we had resolved ourselves to checking with a different neurologist. We had gone to a few very qualified individuals that were open to new avenues of treatment. Some of the medicines were working, and some were making her worse. One medicine in particular really amplified her stress-onset condition. She would have her eyes open and be screaming in pain, writhing on the floor. She told me she could feel everything and that it hurt like hell. These types of episodes were very unsettling. We found out about the medicine by trying different levels and finally trying other ones. There was another medicine that made her physically unstable, and she was losing her memory if she received any head trauma due to the medicine that made her lose it in the first place.

Having the right doctor with an open mind that will actually tailor the treatment to the patient without prejudice is a very important part of solving the problem. When multiple dosages and combinations have no effect, it is time to switch gears to a new treatment. You have to see a good correlation of treatment to positive response. When there is only a worsening negative trend, you aren't in the right ballpark. My wife was a long-term Monte Carlo test [a test that uses repeated sampling to determine a result] of almost all medicines available for epilepsy. A combinational chemistry study was what was occurring. The number of possibilities was staggering. When she changed doctors, it was a bumpy ride. She was given a class of medicine that caused her stress seizures to get a lot worse. She would be screaming, locked in a conscious, self-contained pain spasm that could not be stopped.

Fortunately, we found a neurologist who worked with us and knew enough about the medicine to guide us down a path of treatment that avoided a lot of the problems and put my wife on a path to recovery. She has been seizure/spell-free for over seven months now, and we are grateful. In all of this, she had only lost her will to fight once; then she got back on her feet and kept a positive attitude after that, which eventually resulted in her being able to lead a healthy, functional life. Now she enriches my life every day. Thank you to all who have made that possible.

99

Person with PNES, Australia

I was diagnosed with conversion disorder—another name for non-epileptic seizures—in September 2012 when I was diagnosed with breast cancer. I have had seizures every single day since. I have learned that I have no control of them. I don't know from day to day why I get them or when I'm going to get them. I do know that my subconscious is thinking about something, and when it has thought about something too much, then I have a seizure. I unfortunately don't get any warning; I just have to mentally get on with things so that it doesn't get me too depressed.

100

Person with PNES, UK

I began having seizures when I was sixteen, after I was removed from my mother's care by social services. I thought they were panic attacks, and it wasn't until I mentioned it to my mental health doctor that they referred me to hospital for a sleep-deprived EEG. It came back as generalized idiopathic epilepsy, but after another EEG, a neurologist said that it was a side effect of my bipolar disorder, there was nothing I could do, and I was discharged.

It wasn't until I moved to a different city and my seizures were becoming very frequent, some occasionally lasting over an hour, that my general practitioner referred me to the neurology department there. That neurologist was shocked that the previous one had suggested it was a side effect of bipolar disorder. He said I was having non-epileptic and epileptic seizures and started me on an anti-epileptic drug, which unfortunately didn't help the seizures and made me very depressed. I had another EEG and an MRI, which came back with no epileptic activity. When I went back for a review, they discontinued my tablets and said that my seizures were non-epileptic and that they believed them to be an effect of post-traumatic stress disorder. The neurologist discharged me and referred me to somewhere that specializes in non-epileptic disorders. I've been on the waiting list for about eight months now, but have still heard nothing.

My last seizure was last week at work, when it was quite hot and I was feeling anxious; fortunately, it didn't last long. Currently I am having one or two a week. I think they increase when I'm stressed or upset.

101

Person with PNES, UK

I have lived with non-epileptic seizures for the past six months. This may not seem like a long time to the outside world, but for me, so much has changed during this time. When I have a seizure, there are never any significant triggers or causes. They are unexpected, and therefore I am unable to prepare the surrounding people or myself. One common theme throughout my attacks is that either my wrist or ankle will begin to slightly twitch before I experience a full seizure. During the seizure, I will shake and jerk uncontrollably. My eyes are closed, sharpening my other senses (i.e., my hearing). Occasionally, I will cry in anger during my attacks as I am aware of what is happening; I am just failing to control it and unable to respond. There have been times during attacks that I have seen and heard things that are not actually there and have had to be reassured by surrounding people that I am in a safe environment. My seizures can either be singular, lasting for up to five minutes, or I can have cluster seizures, which will be short bouts of thirty seconds repeated. The after effects of my attacks can vary widely, from tiredness and fatigue to changes in my memory and speech. However, the most common after effect for me is the changes in my mental state as they leave me in an extremely low mood with thoughts of self-harm and overdose.

The first time I suffered an attack, I was in a lecture hall with over two hundred other students. As you can imagine, a university lecture hall is daunting enough for any person but especially for me; I was petrified. As the lecture on psychology went on, I began to feel extremely warm and clammy, my anxiety levels rising by the minute. With my legs constantly tapping and my pen repeatedly clicking, I began irritating my fellow students; that's when she noticed, my best friend. She sat beside me each and every day, and that day was no exception. She looked after me after I was taken out of the lecture hall. She stayed with me and supported me while I was slipping in and out of consciousness, and she held my hand all the way to the hospital. I am lucky to have had her as a friend. However, my condition has taken its toll on our friendship as I no longer attend university with her, and I am not comfortable in a lot of other public places as I worry that I may suffer an attack. I have lots of people to thank for looking after me on that day, from university staff to my best friend and boyfriend as well as the paramedic team.

Non-epileptic seizures have an underestimated effect on a person's daily life; an extremely relevant example of this for me can be seen in my relationships with others. As a university student, I had moved out of my childhood home into halls of residence in which I shared a flat with five other students. I never regretted this decision to move out. I loved having more independence, but I regularly went home on weekends to see my family. My condition has taken this away from me as it has been strongly advised for me to move back home into a more stable environment. Although I have a predominately positive relationship with my family, this has caused strain between us because although they are supportive, I feel as though they now do not trust me in fear that I may have an attack. I also have two younger siblings who I have become isolated from. In my parents view, I set a bad example— "You don't want to grow up like your sister." On the other hand, my boyfriend has been extremely supportive throughout the whole time I have been struggling with my attacks. Being epileptic himself, he is very knowledgeable about how to look after me when my attacks do occur and how to support me to recover emotionally as well as physically.

Only a few weeks ago, I suffered my first attack at my newest place of employment. Before this attack, I got on well with all of my work colleagues both in and out of uniform. However, now that they have seen an attack of my non-epileptic disorder, they have smothered me, constantly asking if I am "okay" and if I am feeling well enough to work. Some may see this as caring; however, for me, with this condition, it irritates me why people treat me differently. They all say that they are there for me if I ever need anything, but in reality, they are only saying that to make themselves feel better.

I thought doctors and nurses were there to help you. In my experience, they have been very dismissive of my condition. It is as if once I had my EEG results saying that my seizures are not caused by an electrical abnormality in my brain, I was no longer a priority. They seemed to stop caring about my health and focused more on what tablets they could use to stop me calling the surgery ["doctor's surgery" is where general practitioners see patients]. Once I had been referred to neurology at the hospital, things started looking up. I was quickly referred to the psychotherapy department; however, I do not fit their criteria for treatment as I was too "unstable." I once again felt as though I had been left alone to fight this battle.

As previously mentioned, I have lost most forms of independence as I have once again been taken under my parents' wing like when I was a child. Furthermore, after suffering my first attack at university, I was removed from my studies as I am deemed to be "unfit to study." Both these elements were and still are extremely important to me as they are major steps in laying out the foundations of my future career. Having these taken away from me as a result of my condition is frustrating and debilitating because I feel as though I am no longer capable of reaching my career goals. In addition, following my first and only attack to date at work, my hours of employment have been cut substantially; my manager feels as though I could benefit from more rest and less responsibility. This alone is infuriating. I thoroughly enjoyed working as it kept my mind busy and active, but now I am stuck at home feeling even more cut off from the world than before. Sometimes I really hate what this condition is doing to my life. I feel so small in the big wide world; it's as if I am alone fighting this battle. Not only has my condition affected my physical health, but also my mental health.

Prior to suffering from non-epileptic attack disorder, I had been diagnosed with chronic panic disorder, which is also severely debilitating as I suffer from recurrent unexpected panic attacks. Much like non-epileptic attack disorder, this condition is less talked about and, in my opinion, is not treated equally alongside many other physical illnesses. Combined, these disorders make my day-to-day life very worrying. There is no trigger for my particular case, so it is hard to say what not to do and what to avoid, leading to great uncertainty and increasing isolation. Not only has my non-epileptic attack disorder changed the way I feel about myself, but it has also changed the way people view me as a person. My parents and my family see me as much more needy; however, it is they that feel the need to take my independence away as a matter of safety. My work colleagues and university staff see me as incapable of work and responsibility. But my highly supportive boyfriend sees me as stronger than ever given that I am fighting this, trying to get better, and doing everything it takes. Like they say, there are two sides to every coin.

Before being initially diagnosed, the doctors and other medical staff referred to it as "pseudoseizures." At first I thought they were calling me a liar, as if I had made it all up! It made me feel as though I had wasted their time and in fact there was nothing wrong with me, but as my disorder developed, they began to see a pattern, which led to testing. During the testing phase, I remember wishing that I had epilepsy just so people would actually take me seriously and I could be treated. Non-epileptic attack disorder cannot be thoroughly explained to each individual patient because it may not be possible to determine a direct cause or trigger. It also can vary massively between cases as there is too much variance to quantify. I have failed to start treatment to help me manage or reduce my non-epileptic attacks because I failed to meet the criteria to receive psychotherapy. So, at the moment, I am attempting to carry on with my non-independent, smothered life as best as possible. Compared to when I was first diagnosed, my perspective on my disorder is more positive; I have learned to cope with my attacks and have accepted that they are now a part of my life.

102

Person with PNES, Israel

PART 1: INTERNALIZED ABLEISM*

"Help! Help!"

"Wait. I can help myself."

I move my right arm an inch to the left. Finally. I intended to move it away from being locked under my back, but it wouldn't move farther. I fell with my arm in that position. That's one of the weird things about seizures. Your body may twist and turn in ways you don't imagine you could move in.

Then the convulsions start again.

"You can do this. You can! Stop convulsing! Now! The doctor said it is psychological, so if you really want it to stop it will."

I continue seizing. My arms convulse, and my legs are locked in a ramrod straight position.

"See? This is the work of your inner child. You must work through the abuse. It is making you sick."

Exhausted, I let out a long breath. My legs are getting some movement back, and my arms have stopped convulsing. Finally. I inhale deeply.

"You can do this. I know you can. You are strong. Resilient. Powerful. No seizure can overtake you."

"But it is overtaking me." And I finally let out the long-awaited cry. "It is. I can't stop it. There must be something medically wrong with me. Why do the doctors keep saying it's my anxiety? My post-traumatic stress disorder? I'm not even anxious now!"

Nothing makes sense, and everything is spinning. My entire life as I knew it dramatically changed, and I am left with an average of fifty seizures a day.

* Ableism is like racism but towards people with disability.

Doctors tell me it's my anxiety, and I know as much as anyone that I get panic attacks constantly. Could it be that? It must be. That and the trauma are the only answers I am getting.

PART 2: IT IS NOT JUST PSYCHOLOGICAL

Something wasn't right. My psychiatrists say that I have all these symptoms because of trauma. But I worked through the trauma intensively. After three years of intensive therapy and six months in a psychiatric outpatient program, my post-traumatic stress disorder has decreased a lot. I thoroughly worked through the abuse. Mentally, I feel like a changed person. My anxiety is way lower, and my panic attacks are down to once a week instead of throughout the day. Something doesn't add up. If trauma was making me sick, why weren't my physical symptoms getting better instead of becoming worse while my psychological ones were decreasing?

I believe that there is something more to the physiology of conversion disorder that scientists are missing. This isn't just trauma based. There is either a permanent change in my brain, this is a multidisciplinary disease, or they are missing something else.

As I scrolled the internet for answers, I came across a spiritual healer who uses hypnosis. Medicine gave me no answers. Psychology gave me no answers. Maybe she would have them. And she did.

PART 3: PAST LIVES

The chills ran through me, through and through. No. I do not want to believe in past lives. Especially if it has to do with me. This stuff is creepy. It haunts me. No! I am absolutely not going to believe that my seizures are caused by traumas from past lives.

I inhale deeply and look at the facts. Repetitive dreams with the same storyline that bewilder me. Where did they come from? Then these strange unfamiliar, seizures where I fall in a position I have never fallen in before. During those seizures, something pulled at my heart. It felt emotional. My body was telling me something, yet I didn't know what it was. I knew there was more to the story. When I saw the hypnotist, the process brought me back to another lifetime where I had been traumatized and fallen in the exact same position as I have in my strange seizures.

It would be so easy to ignore the recovered memory. I could throw it away in a wishy-washy, this-isn't-concrete sort of way. Everything inside me begged me not to believe this. But it made so much sense. Months of the same nightmares. The seizures where I clearly knew my body was telling me a story but I didn't know what it was. The traumatic memory where I had fallen in the exact same position.

I reached out to two women who had seen this hypnotist for fibromyalgia and come out completely healed. I asked them question after question for a full hour. And they too had a trauma of past lives that made them sick. And when they did a healing process with this practitioner, they completely recovered. I believed them. These people weren't lying. If past lives could cause them physical illness, why couldn't it be the same for me?

I submit to the truth glaring me in the face. My conversion disorder is not just from current life trauma, but from past lives as well.

PART 4: STEPPING INTO FREEDOM

Working through the trauma from past lives is a process I am still in. All I can say is that I am doing tremendously better mentally, physically, and emotionally with it. It feels like I have stepped into freedom. I am so much happier, lighter, and filled with much zest for life.

I still believe that conversion disorder is a multidisciplinary disease or that there is a lot more to the neuropsychiatric component than we are currently aware of.

I don't believe that past life trauma is affecting every person with a conversion disorder. Not at all. Nor do I believe that every person with this disorder has gone through a huge traumatic event. It has been said that even small and seemingly insignificant stressful events can cause trauma if our brain does not process the event properly. Many times, trauma is a factor with conversion disorder.

Eventually, with time and a compassionate therapist, I learned to be compassionate to myself and how the internalized ableism and rough manner I thought to myself during seizures that were destructive for my overall well-being.

Now the thoughts during my seizures look like this:

"Honey, it's okay. You're going to be okay. I love you. I want you to know that. No seizure, no disability, no ableism toward you takes away from your self-worth. This is so hard honey, I know. I don't want you to suffer so. I love you."

This dramatic change freed me beyond any measure. I am now much less anxious about having seizures around people, and I know that even if people will be mean and abusive toward me, then at least I will be kind to myself.

103

Person with PNES, USA

My story starts a few years ago, in 2012. I was working overnight shifts at a big box retailer, and it was an incredibly stressful job. Things outside of work were stressful, but they were going fairly well. I started having spells of minor confusion after which I would sleep for the day. That went on for about three months before I had my first discovered seizure. My first seizure occurred in my sleep and was discovered by my wife. Her mother has epilepsy, so she had seen several seizures before my own. She tried to convince me to go to the doctor, but I would not go at first. I had another seizure before too long, though, and decided to reach out to my primary care physician at the time.

Being only twenty-five, my primary care physician had told me that there was no way I had a seizure. He had stated that he thought it was all in my head "because people my age do not just start having seizures for no reason." Turns out that I had fallen and knocked myself out about a year prior. I had slipped on some ice in my mother's driveway and do not know how long I was unconscious. I did not seek medical attention at the time because I did not seem to have any issues, just a simple lump on the back of my head as if I had bumped it on something. I did not even experience any symptoms that would have indicated a mild concussion.

Progress a few months forward, and I had managed to make contact with a new neurologist at a local medical facility. He immediately placed me on an anti-epileptic drug. I had an MRI and EEG performed. After a few months, I had an additional seizure, and my medication was increased. Three months later, another seizure and another medication boost. I held out for about six to eight months on the high dose before I had another cluster of seizures. My medication was increased even more. A few more months and a few more seizures later, my medication was adjusted to an even higher dose. I maintained on this dose for about a year before trouble decided to rear up again.

About two and a half years after I had my first seizure, I was up to the maximum dose of the anti-epileptic drug that I was on and was having seizures at a greater frequency. There are many days that I do not remember. I had difficulty maintaining focus and started needing greater amounts of sleep to get through the day. I was dragging through my work, and many facets of my life were suffering.

About mid-2014, my biological father had passed away. A few months later, my adopted father had been diagnosed with a very aggressive case of small cell lung cancer. He was also diagnosed with dermatomyositis, which had started to affect his mind and ability to function. He was gone by January of 2015. My adopted mother passed a few months later in May of 2015, and I lost my job that same week from a combination of absences due to my seizures growing to about three occurrences per month and the stress of losing loved ones. My life was falling apart, and it seemed like I was just drowning in sorrow and my own illness. I contemplated suicide on a regular basis, but I just couldn't bring myself to do that to my wife and my friends. I knew nothing would get better if I just gave up.

I spent six weeks out of work before I was to find another job in a computer parts warehouse. Things were barely holding together, and I had to file bankruptcy due to the combined pile of medical bills and personal bills. About six months into this new job, I fell into what seemed to be a nearly endless loop of seizures. We tried several different medications to work in tandem with the anti-epileptic drug, and nothing seemed to help or the side effects were worse than the seizures. I checked with a different neurologist at the same medical facility who simply threw a few more medications my way. Once I had a severe allergic reaction to a new anti-epileptic drug that I was given and could not take it any longer. I was missing an average of two days per week at my job due to having seizures. My new primary care physician decided to send me to a specialized medical center at a department of neurology.

I met with my new neurologist who had decided that something was not right with my current treatment. After evaluating my situation, it was deemed best that I spend some time under a monitored EEG study. All medication was ceased, and I spent six days hooked up to an EEG monitor. In that week, we were only able to monitor a single seizure. To have stopped the medication abruptly, and to have not had any seizures, was a big eye opener for me. I was not being treated for the correct problem! We had determined at this point that I did not have partial complex epilepsy as previously diagnosed. It was discovered that I have non-epileptic seizures. We have narrowed several things down and determined that stress and larger quantities of caffeine tend to cause me to be much more prone to having a seizure.

Shortly after my stay at the medical center and the complete overhaul of my medication, I lost my job again. I had been doing well and having fewer and fewer seizures, but I was still missing work here and there because of them. I found a new job working hospitality at one of the major hotel chains. And with some tweaking of my new treatment, I was able to function almost as if nothing was wrong. I then found employment at a much higher paying job and tried working hospitality at the hotel as a part-time job. I had been trying to rebound from the financial collapse I suffered in 2015, but it seemed that my seizures would have no part of it. Working both jobs was causing me to begin having seizures again. I also began having panic attacks at this point. I lost the higher paying job and was fortunate enough that the other still had a full-time position available.

I have been working full-time and do not currently have health insurance. Because of the seizures and panic attacks, I have not been able to hold down a job that has insurance that I can afford. The non-epileptic seizures have made my life quite difficult, but I keep rolling forward. There have been some serious bouts of depression for me to fight through, but so far, I continue to come out on top of them. There is still a great feeling of fear that stays with me, though, because I am afraid that more seizures will come and ruin what I have managed to rebuild of my life. My coordination, memory, and learning capacity have been diminished from what I have been through. The stress and all of the different medications that I have been on have taken their toll on my mind.

104

Person with Epilepsy and PNES, UK

I had been a lorry [truck] driver for many years. At the age of forty-two, following the need to close our business, we relocated. In 1982, I had a vasectomy, and after coming home from the hospital and within hours of my operation, I had blackouts and strange dizzy feelings. My doctor at the time diagnosed me with hypoglycemia and told me to take more sugar. I slowly improved but was left with the occasional buzzing sensation and dizzy spells.

In 1988, my wife was fed up with me having to work so many nights away, so I got a job with a local business and relocated nearer to the job. I was still getting dizzy spells, which gradually got worse, and after some months, I started to get pins and needles in my feet. This would then spread up my legs, and I would also get it in my hands and arms. After a while the dizziness would set in, and on several occasions I passed out. I was taken to the hospital, where they did blood tests and told me that my blood sugars were okay and that I had probably fainted. I saw another doctor near my new home who thought it might be caused by the strain from heavy lifting and signed me off work for three months. During this time, I saw a specialist at another hospital who thought it might be narcolepsy. The dizziness continued, and my doctor signed me off for another three months and thought I might be suffering from depression.

I became very fed up with being at home, and in 1990, I started back at work at a local service station on nights but continued to collapse at times. During this time I saw my doctor again, who said that I could be suffering from stress due to lack of sleep. I changed my job again and went back to driving, but without the heavy lifting. However, this meant long journeys and early starts. I was okay for a while, but then the dizziness came back and I was stopping so that I could sleep several times a day as this seemed to help. I started to get the pins and needles sensation more often, and my wife suggested that I see the doctor again, who this time thought it might be hyperventilation.

After this I was driving locally, and one day when I went to overtake [pass] a slow-moving car, everything came back, including the dizziness and the buzzing sensation. I had to stop on the wrong side of the road and get out of the cab. My legs gave way, and I was crawling around on my hands and knees. I thought I was going to pass out and felt badly disorientated.

Although I had never told anyone, I had experienced this strong sensation a couple of times before. On June 7, 1993, I had a long trip south. I started at 2:30 in the morning; the day became very hot. I had completed about four deliveries and was heading for the Mail Sorting Office. I had stopped several times for a sleep because of feeling odd, and when I arrived at the sorting office, I made my delivery. I remember starting to drive out of the yard, but the next thing I knew, I was waking up at a T-junction/intersection. It was like the lights had gone out in my head. I then started to hear voices. These voices were soft at first, but then they became more and more clear and were reassuring. Then the lights came back on, and when I finally awoke, there was an ambulance crew talking to me. I was very, very frightened because I did not remember how I got there, let alone how I had managed to stop the lorry. The crew of the ambulance wanted me to go to the hospital with them, but I was very confused, disorientated, and scared, so I said, "No." Then I started the vehicle up. They said that if I drove off they would inform the police and get me picked up, but I drove off anyway in a panic. I didn't know where I was going, I just thought that eventually I would come across a signpost and get my bearings. I decided to go back without going on the motorways as that is where the police would probably be looking for me. I just had to get home to my wife. On the way back, I made one more delivery, and everything was fine, the strange sensation had gone. However, my employer had phoned me on the mobile, and he couldn't understand anything I said, so although I thought I was okay, I obviously wasn't. Evidently he was extremely worried about me, but I only found that out later. I found myself on the motorway and all was well until I got to the next junction. I then pulled out to overtake again, and it all came back. I froze at the wheel. I was petrified and in a state of panic, and I couldn't move my hands to turn the steering wheel. My body went rigid, and I had no control over it. I was stuck in the middle lane. I started to reduce speed. and vehicles behind me were flashing their lights at me. Then everything went blank until I found myself back in the state I was in earlier. I started to get my senses back, the sound of traffic got slowly stronger, and then I was awake. Somehow, I don't know how, I found that I had moved over and was driving in the emergency lane. (Was there such a thing as a guardian angel looking after me, taking over the driving when I passed out?)

I had experienced the strange feelings again, but this time, I had passed out at the wheel, bitten my tongue, and come to be covered in blood. The next day following this, I went to see my general practitioner, who diagnosed epilepsy. He told me that I would have to surrender my driving license, which meant I lost my job. There was no help or advice given. My wife and I were left to just get on with it.

Shortly after this, my family and I went on holiday, and during the journey, I had to keep getting out of the car and walk around to get rid of the strange sensations. Shortly after arriving, I had more and more episodes. These got so bad that my wife called a local general practitioner, who dialed 999 [the emergency number for the UK], and an ambulance arrived to take me to the hospital. During the journey there, the episodes worsened, and I passed out and stopped breathing for a short while; I also developed jerking movements. The ambulance crew diverted to the nearest hospital, where I was told that I had had grand mal seizures and the consultant started me on an anti-epileptic drug. The journey home was equally traumatic, and the moment we arrived, my wife called our general practitioner, who prescribed a relaxant to help.

The epilepsy medication, however, produced side effects, and I was put on several types, eventually settling on one. This stopped the grand mal seizures. However, I still experienced the weird sensations (that I was told were complex partial seizures) several times a week. This was the start of many hospital visits over the next two decades for my epilepsy, including CT scans, MRIs, and two ambulatory EEGs. I got to the point where I was prescribed several anti-epileptic drugs. Some of these add-ons had a dire effect on my mental state and caused psychotic episodes. I was zombie-like and experiencing an ever-increasing issue with my short- and long-term memory. None of the medications stopped the partial seizures, which manifested themselves as screaming phrases like "No, no, no!" or "Stop, stop, stop!" I sometimes cried profusely or laughed when there was nothing to laugh at. I would fall to the floor and scream for help, holding on to anything at hand for dear life, every time thinking that I was going to die. I hated the intense fear generated by these seizures. Sometimes I experienced a change in mood and knew that a seizure was going to happen, but other times the onset was sudden with no warning. Some days my thinking was just so slow that I couldn't do even the simplest of tasks unaided. I nearly always slept after a seizure. They often came in clusters, increasing in intensity as they went on. This meant that I was on a high dosage of a relaxant to relieve the symptoms.

Eventually my wife went against the medical advice we were being given and gradually reduced the medication to a small amount. My memory improved a bit, and I felt more like myself. The complex partial seizures continued, however. I could not work and eventually was registered as disabled. The high dosage of drugs affected my balance, and I had serious issues when walking. Because of the level of seizures, I needed carers to look after me when my wife was not around. Apart from a yearly brief visit to a consultant, all investigations into my condition stopped. Life slipped into some sort of routine, and although I could not work for a living, I did manage some voluntary work from home for a charity.

Between 2014 and 2016, I was taken into the hospital three times because my seizures became continuous for a period of twelve hours or more. This prompted my original neurological consultant to look at my case again. On January 3, 2017, I went into a neurological hospital for another set of video telemetry. My medication was removed, and I had numerous seizures that were caught on film. The consultant who diagnosed epilepsy about twenty-five years ago told me that the episodes they witnessed were not epilepsy but dissociative (non-epileptic) seizures. He stated that I have both epilepsy and dissociative seizures. I was prescribed an anti-epileptic drug as it was thought that this may help, but apart from that, there was no other advice or help as to where I might get information about the condition. I was not told about a non-epileptic attack disorder website or any others.

My newly diagnosed dissociative seizures seem to be the same as the old ones. I still cry or get sad and shout repetitive phrases. The intense fear has not gone away, and although I do not get the tingling sensations anymore, the dizziness is still there. However, with the anti-epileptic drug, the effect on my life has altered as I seem to only get the seizures every two to three weeks now, but instead of the usual one or two episodes, I can get them for a whole day at a time.

This condition has meant that I was forced to give up a career that I loved and left me needing twenty-four-hour care and being totally dependent on others. I feel it has ruined the life I had. I am in a state of confusion and wondering where I can go from here and what life now holds for me at the ripe old age of seventy-two.

105

Person with PNES, USA

I had back surgery in 2013. I went in as an emergency patient and was kept on bed rest for nearly two weeks. I was told that I might end up paralyzed because of the area of damage to my spine. Recovery from surgery was slow and difficult. While I was at home healing, I developed a stutter. Then I began noticing uncontrolled twitching in my fingers and hands. The twitching progressed to jerking of my muscles. The main areas affected were my arms, hands, and shoulders. However, I did experience seizures in my legs, face, and torso.

After an EEG followed by a video-EEG, it was determined that my seizures were of the psychogenic non-epileptic variety. This was a lot to absorb. After researching it a bit, I was able to see how the diagnosis could be accurate. I was referred to a neuropsychiatrist, and after a couple of visits, the doctor recommended a twelve-week course during which I would meet with him and would have a workbook to complete.

I agreed to this method of treatment but didn't understand how this could benefit me. I was quite skeptical and a bit intimidated at the thought of being seen by a neuropsychiatrist. I did (and do) believe the body and mind are entwined. However, deep down, I was convinced that there was something the doctors were missing in their diagnosis. Certainly, there had to be a test that would show the exact cause of my symptoms.

I began working with the doctor and started seeing how my thought process and how I handled stressors in my life were impacting me in many ways. The seizures were just another signal from my body that something had to change. It was my body's way of showing me that I needed to address the psychological pain I was experiencing.

He made it clear early on that I would be going through this training for myself and nobody else. He told me that I would get out of it only as much as I put in. I decided to place it at the top of my priority list as much as I could. I read every chapter at least twice and tried to apply what I was learning. I wasn't always as successful as I wanted, but every week I became healthier and better able to sort out my thoughts and feelings. I learned to be more honest and assertive in my communication. I let go of much of the heavy load of anxiety that I had carried for as long as I can remember. My seizures became less and less a part of my daily life.

The doctor taught me how to use the tools that I need to carry on and be more in control of my own thoughts and actions and, consequently, more in control of my seizures. I learned to use thought records to sort out my negative thought process. He showed me a way to breathe deeply and relax. Treatment also involved written homework, keeping a journal and a seizure log. I would track my seizures, noting the time of day, duration of seizure, what was going on when it occurred, and how severe it was.

Time has passed, and life has remained complicated. I would like to say that I have had no seizures since I completed the treatment. I would like to say that I have maintained a relaxed state, free of anxiety. I can't say that, but what I can say is that I have a better handle on managing my symptoms and my life. Seizures are rare, and when they do happen, I am not frightened and don't give in to them. I take a deep breath, reminding myself that I don't need to do that anymore. I examine my thought process and try to dig into what is bothering me. I turn my "self talk" into a more realistic truth. I am so thankful I was able to receive this treatment, and I recommend it to anyone who is experiencing seizures that have been determined to be non-epileptic in nature.

USEFUL CONTACTS

Information about non-epileptic seizures
   www.nonepilepticattacks.info
Web forum and information about non-epileptic seizures
   www.nonepilepticattackdisorder.org.uk
Information about non-epileptic seizures in children and young people
   www.neurokid.co.uk
Information about non-epileptic seizures and other functional neurological
symptoms in many languages
   www.neurosymptoms.org
Information about PNES in French
   www.lareponsedupsy.info/CPNE
Web forum and information about functional neurological disorder
   www.fndaction.org.uk
Web forum and information about functional neurological disorder
   www.fndhope.org
Epilepsy Action
   www.epilepsy.org.uk
Epilepsy Foundation of America
   www.epilepsy.com
Epilepsy Scotland
   www.epilepsyscotland.org.uk
Epilepsy Society
   www.epilepsysociety.org.uk
National Institutes of Health
   www.ninds.nih.gov/Disorders/All-Disorders/Epilepsy-Information-
   Page
Northeast Regional Epilepsy Group
   www.epilepsygroup.com
Samaritans
   www.samaritans.org

INDEX

abdominal seizures, 30, 33

ableism, internalized, 245–46

absence seizures, 90, 92, 99, 158, 203
  characteristics of, xiii, 91, 174–75, 196, 210–11
  descriptions and experiences of, 52, 99, 211
  diagnosis of, 91, 196
  triggers of, 91

abuse, xiv, 17, 50, 70, 73, 87, 120, 162, 233, 245, 246. *See also* child abuse; sexual abuse; trauma

Accident and Emergency Department, 12, 21, 40, 91, 117–19, 123, 129, 155, 167, 178–79, 196
  negative experiences in, 66–67, 96–97, 118, 119, 179, 202, 203, 206–7
  reluctance to go to, 66, 91

acupuncture, 155–56

AIDS, 115, 116

air purifiers, 231

alcohol abuse, 115, 202

alcohol intoxication
  seizure patients appearing drunk, 194
  seizure patients suspected of, 39, 174, 177, 197

alcohol use by seizure patients
  abstinence from, 62, 165
  attitudes regarding, 39–40
  seizures caused or worsened by, 39, 40, 62

allergic reactions to medications, 106, 140, 249

allergies, 65, 67, 142, 231. *See also* asthma

allergy medications, 142

alone, being. *See* home; loneliness; social isolation

alternative medicine, 58, 113, 115, 137, 224, 235. *See also* cannabis

ambulance crews/ambulance staff, 13, 66, 118–20, 167. *See also* paramedics

ambulances, 40, 43, 57, 66, 192, 221, 252

ambulance technicians. *See* emergency medical technicians

amnesia. *See* blackouts; memory lapses; memory loss

animals, service. *See* dogs: guide

anti-anxiety drugs. *See* anxiolytics

anticonvulsants. *See* anti-epileptic drugs; anti-seizure medications

antidepressants, 35, 36, 43, 54, 65, 96, 109, 116, 128, 137, 140, 141, 147, 167, 184
  improvement following use of, 228, 232
  postpartum, 190

anti-epileptic drugs, 90, 91, 118, 142, 193, 206, 249, 253. *See also* anti-seizure medications; *specific topics*
  high doses, 89, 248
  low doses, 106, 142
  mood stabilization from, 175, 193
  negative reactions to, 106, 249
  side effects, 90, 253
  stopping/getting off, 29, 76, 89, 143, 225, 228, 249, 254 (*see also* withdrawal syndrome from medications)

anti-seizure medications, 33, 161, 167. *See also* anti-epileptic drugs

anxiety, 109, 210. *See also* fear; panic
  as cause of seizures, 52, 99, 109, 141, 142, 144, 147, 149, 245, 246
  history of, 10, 12, 61, 65, 89, 147
  interventions for, 142 (*see also* anxiolytics)
  prior to seizure, 91, 109

anxiety disorders, 10, 83, 108, 111, 140–41, 181. *See also* anxiety; anxiolytics; panic attacks